EMQs for the MRCOG Part 2

EMQs for the MRCOG Part 2
A self-assessment guide

Kalaivani Ramalingam DGO MRCOG
Specialist Registrar
Obstetrics and Gynaecology
Princess Anne Hospital
Southampton
UK

Latha M Palanivelu DGO MRCOG
Registrar
Obstetrics and Gynaecology
Milton Keynes General Hospital
Milton Keynes
UK

Jeremy Brockelsby BSc MB BS PhD MRCOG
Consultant in Feto-Maternal Medicine
Addenbrooke's Hospital
Cambridge University NHS Foundation Trust
Cambridge
UK

Christian Phillips DM MRCOG
Consultant Obstetrician and Gynaecologist
Basingstoke and North Hampshire Foundation Trust Hospital
Basingstoke
UK

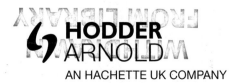

HODDER ARNOLD
AN HACHETTE UK COMPANY

First published in Great Britain in 2008 by
Hodder Arnold, an imprint of Hodder Education, an Hachette UK Company,
338 Euston Road, London NW1 3BH

http://www.hoddereducation.com

Whilst the advice and information in this book are believed to be true and
accurate at the date of going to press, neither the authors nor the publisher
can accept any legal responsibility or liability for any errors or omissions
that may be made. In particular, (but without limiting the generality of the
preceding disclaimer) every effort has been made to check drug dosages;
however it is still possible that errors have been missed. Furthermore,
dosage schedules are constantly being revised and new side-effects
recognized. For these reasons the reader is strongly urged to consult the
drug companies' printed instructions before administering any of the drugs
recommended in this book.

British Library Cataloguing in Publication Data
A catalogue record for this book is available from the British Library

Library of Congress Cataloging-in-Publication Data
A catalog record for this book is available from the Library of Congress

ISBN- 978-0-340-941690

3 4 5 6 7 8 9 10

Commissioning Editor:	Gavin Jamieson
Project Editor:	Francesca Naish
Production Controller:	Andre Sim
Cover Design:	Helen Townson
Indexer:	Laurence Errington

Typeset in 10/12 Minion by Charon Tec Ltd (A Macmillan Company),
Chennai, India
Printed in India

What do you think about this book? Or any other Hodder Arnold title?
Please visit our website: www.hoddereducation.com

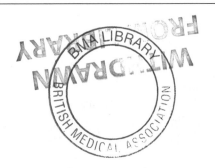

Contents

Foreword   viii
Preface   ix

Introduction   x

Section 1: General obstetrics   **1**
  Questions   2
    1 Advanced life support   2
    2 Medicolegal issues   3
  Answers   4

Section 2: Operative obstetrics   **6**
  Questions   7
    3 Caesarean section   7
    4 Obstetric anaesthesia   8
    5 Delivery room management   9
  Answers   10

Section 3: Medical complications   **12**
  Questions   13
    6 Breast cancer in pregnancy   13
    7 Infections in pregnancy   14
    8 Perinatal infection   15
    9 HIV infections in pregnancy   16
   10 Obstetric cholestasis   17
   11 Management of abdominal pain in pregnancy   19
   12 Diagnosis of abdominal pain in pregnancy   20
   13 Gastrointestinal disorders in pregnancy   22
   14 Thromboembolism/venous disorders   23
   15 Syncope in pregnancy   24
   16 Thyroid diseases complicating pregnancy   25
   17 Chest pain in pregnancy   27
   18 Diabetes in pregnancy   29
   19 Palpitations in pregnancy   30
   20 Vomiting/liver function tests in pregnancy   31
   21 Medications in pregnancy   33
   22 Psychiatric disorders in pregnancy and the puerperium 34

CONTENTS

23 Headache   35
Answers   36

Section 4: Labour and puerperium   **49**
Questions   50
24 Mechanism of labour   50
25 Third-stage complications   51
26 Intrapartum care   52
27 Maternal collapse   54
28 Shoulder dystocia   55
29 Postpartum haemorrhage   56
30 Intrauterine death   57
31 Preterm labour   58
32 Perineal injuries   59
33 Malpresentations   60
34 Labour risks   61
35 Tests on the labour suite   62
Answers   63

Section 5: Antenatal care   **72**
Questions   73
36 Antenatal screening   73
37 Genetics   74
38 Large for dates   75
Answers   76

Section 6: Benign gynaecological conditions   **78**
Questions   79
39 Vulval ulcers   79
40 Management of fibroids   80
41 Uterovaginal prolapse   81
42 Müllerian defects   82
43 Management of menorrhagia   83
44 Cervical screening   84
45 Gestational trophoblastic disease   85
46 Paediatric gynaecology   86
Answers   87

Section 7: Gynaecological oncology   **93**
Questions   94
47 Management of endometrial cancer   94
48 Treatment of cervical cancer   96
49 Vulval carcinoma   97
50 Management of adnexal mass   98
51 Colposcopy   99
Answers   100

CONTENTS

Section 8: Surgical gynaecology   **104**
Questions   105
    52   Postoperative period investigations   105
    53   Management of postoperative complications   107
    54   Urinary tract injuries   108
    55   Late postoperative complications   109
Answers   110

Section 9: Subfertility   **114**
Questions   115
    56   Management of subfertility   115
    57   Causes of subfertility   117
    58   Investigation of amenorrhoea   119
Answers   120

Section 10: Urogynaecology   **123**
Questions   124
    59   Diagnosis of urinary conditions   124
    60   Management options in urogynaecology   125
Answers   126

Section 11: Menopause and HRT   **128**
Questions   129
    61   Postmenopausal bleeding   129
    62   Choice of HRT   131
    63   Choice of HRT   132
Answers   133

Section 12: Sexual health and contraception   **136**
Questions   137
    64   Human immunodeficiency virus infection   137
    65   Choice of contraception   138
    66   Emergency contraception   139
    67   Contraception   140
    68   Termination of pregnancy   141
    69   Sexually transmitted infections   142
Answers   144

Section 13: Early pregnancy complications   **149**
Questions   150
    70   Recurrent miscarriage   150
    71   Management of bleeding in early pregnancy   151
Answers   152

Index   **155**

Foreword

There has been an increasing emphasis on education and assessment in medical schools and postgraduate institutions during the past 20 years, with many changes introduced into teaching and assessment methods for the student and trainee. It is generally acknowledged that assessments often direct and drive learning, and it is therefore vital that the content of the assessment reflects the learning objectives.

The extended matching question (EMQ), a form of multiple choice question (MCQ), was introduced in the early 1990s to overcome some of the criticisms levelled at unidimensional multiple choice question, by testing factual and applied knowledge. The extended list of offered options or potential answers (15, as here, being considered an ideal number) reduces the opportunity for students to guess the correct answers as conventional MCQs allow; EMQs are more discriminating and result in a greater spread of marks with consequent improved reliability. Importantly, they maintain the advantage of allowing computerised marking, with consequent savings in time and manpower.

EMQs are now used in many medical schools and Royal Colleges, and in 2006 the Royal College of Obstetricians and Gynaecologists introduced this assessment format into the membership examinations. Therefore *EMQs for the MRCOG Part 2* is a timely text that will assist not only those being taught and in training, but also those who are engaged in teaching, by providing guidance and preparation for answering and authoring such questions. Dr Ramalingam and her colleagues have produced a very useful handbook for trainees preparing to sit the College membership examinations; it will be equally resonant with undergraduates preparing for their final examinations in obstetrics and gynaecology. They have selected between one and 16 different themes for each of 11 specialist areas in obstetrics and gynaecology, concentrating on aetiology, diagnosis, investigation or management topics, and providing simple logical explanations for the correct answers for each of the four or five vignettes outlined. They have shown how it is possible to pose a large number of questions based on the same theme or subject area, allowing the questions to be used in more than one examination paper.

The authors are to be congratulated on producing a most useful and readily readable book that will be of great use to both trainee and teacher alike. I expect this first volume to be followed by subsequent editions, expanding the subject areas and topics to be covered, and introducing new concepts in the design of EMQs as this assessment technique develops further.

I Z MacKenzie
Nuffield Department of Obstetrics and Gynaecology
October 2006

Preface

A new format of questions was introduced from September 2006 for the MRCOG part 2, this new method of examination being called extended matching questions (EMQs). The new EMQ paper has 40 questions and constitutes 15 per cent of the total score in the part 2 MRCOG written examination. This is believed to be a fairer assessment compared with other examination techniques.

This book is aimed to familiarise candidates with the new method of examination and covers most topics in obstetrics, gynaecology and related subjects. There are several themes with four or five clinical scenarios in each theme. Practice in this technique of examination is essential; an hour is allowed to answer the 40 EMQs. This method is likely to replace all multiple choice questions in future examination.

Dr K Ramalingam

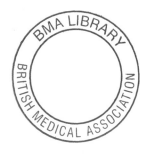

Introduction: An approach to EMQs

This book is written in an attempt to familiarise candidates preparing for part 2 of the MRCOG with the new examination technique. This book is not an alternative for textbooks in preparation for membership examinations, but it is a good companion for doctors preparing for exams.

EMQs are an increasingly popular method to test knowledge on a wider basis. Success in this technique relies on sound knowledge and good time management. The questions are often lengthy and time-consuming to read, which is why candidates have an allotment of 1 hour to answer 40 questions.

Each stem contains 1–5 questions and a maximum of 15 options. A suitable approach will be to read the questions and look for the most appropriate response in the options list. The guidance provided by Royal College of Obstetricians and Gynaecologists confirms that there is no negative marking. More than one response for the same question gains no marks.

An EMQ consists of:

1   a theme;

2   a question (lead-in statement);

3   responses (an option list);

4   problems or clinical situations.

Unlike MCQs, there are many more choices in EMQs. This implies an inability to answer by elimination. The scenario on a topic is more lifelike, making the examination fairer and more as expected in real life.

EMQs are good means for testing out just awareness by application of knowledge. This means more than just recall of factual information. It is objective too as it still has a universal key and is marked by computer. Reliability of scoring is thus maintained in the examination technique.

Research on EMQs has shown that they test good application of knowledge and are excellent in testing the coverage of topics with ease and reliability of scoring. EMQs can be based on the traditional MCQ style, making it mandatory to have factual knowledge to answer such questions. More EMQs are, however, clinical vignettes requiring experience as a registrar/practitioner to be able to approach these questions.

Our suggested method of answering these is to look at the theme and lead-in statement first. After reading each clinical problem, a good candidate must be able to arrive at the answers and look for them in the list of options. Some answers may be factual and straightforward; others may require deduction in terms of the clinical situation or calculations.

Example

Theme: Management of fibroids

Question/lead-in statement: For each of the clinical scenarios choose the best option from the list given below. Each response may be used once, more than once or not at all.

Responses:

A   total hysterectomy
B   myomectomy with prior gonadotrophin-releasing hormone (GnRH) analogue
C   total abdominal hysterectomy and bilateral salpingo-oophorectomy
D   submucosal resection of the fibroid
E   vaginal hysterectomy
F   antibiotics
G   embolisation
H   GnRH analogue
I   transcervical resection of the endometrium
J   catheterisation and antibiotics
K   Mirena intrauterine system
L   conservative management
M   intravenous fluids and analgesics
N   ultrasound monitoring
O   a GnRH analogue followed by hysterectomy

Clinical situations:

1   A 45-year-old nulliparous woman is being evaluated for inflammatory bowel disease as an inpatient. Ultrasound has shown a 5 cm fundal fibroid and a 3 cm anterior wall fibroid. Her periods are regular, 4–5 days in 30 days. She denies any intermenstrual bleeding. She is up to date with her smears, with normal results.

2   A 36-year-old nulliparous woman is being evaluated for secondary subfertility. She has regular heavy periods lasting for 7 days every month. Ultrasound shows a small submucosal fibroid.

3   A 34-year-old para 1 presents 4 weeks after delivery with vomiting and abdominal pain. She is complaining of vaginal bleeding that started 3 days ago. Her haemoglobin level is 8.8 g/dL. On examination, her uterus is about 18 weeks' size. There is fresh vaginal bleeding. Ultrasound shows an enlarged uterus without any retained products of conception.

4   A 43-year-old patient is admitted with acute urinary retention, fever and dysuria. She recollects having heavy periods for the past few months. On examination there is a central 20-week-size mass.

5   A 40-year-old Afro-Caribbean lady presents to her GP with dysmenorrhoea and heavy periods. Her haemoglobin is 9 g/dL. Ultrasound pelvis shows a 26-week-size uterus with multiple fibroids. What is the appropriate management?

Answers:
L D M J O

L   The incidental finding of a fibroid occurs in up to 30 per cent of women in the reproductive age group. No intervention is required if the fibroid is asymptomatic.
D   Subfertility can be caused by a submucosal fibroid acting as an intrauterine contraceptive device. If other factors are normal, submucosal resection is often considered.
M   Red degeneration of a fibroid commonly occurs in the postpartum period. Hydration and adequate analgesia are the first-line management.
J   Large fibroids cause impaction of the uterus and lead to urinary retention. Obstruction with residual urine could lead to recurrent urinary tract infection.
O   Fibroids causing menorrhagia leading to anaemia are often resistant to conservative measures. Hysterectomy is often required. Prior treatment with GnRH helps in reduction of bleeding and decreases the size of fibroid.

List of references and suggested readings

CEMACH. *Why Mothers Die 2000–2002. The Sixth Report of Confidential Enquiries into Maternal Deaths in the United Kingdom.*

Edmonds DK. *Dewhurst's Textbook of Obstetrics and Gynaecology for Postgraduates*, 6th edn. Oxford: Blackwell Science Publishing, 1999.

James DK, Steer PJ, Weiner CP, Gonik B. *High Risk Pregnancy – Management Options*, 3rd edn. Philadelphia, PA: Saunders, 2005.

Luesley D, Baker P. *Obstetrics and Gynaecology – an Evidence-based Text for MRCOG.* London: Hodder Arnold, 2004.

Nelson-Piercy C. *Handbook of Obstetric Medicine*, 3rd edn. London: Taylor & Francis, 2006.

Royal College of Obstetricians and Gynaecologists. Clinical *Green Top Guidelines*

Royal College of Obstetricians and Gynaecologists. *National Evidence-Based Clinical Guidelines.*

Shaw RW, Soutter WP, Stanton SL. *Gynaecology*, 3rd edn. Edinburgh: Churchill Livingstone, 2003.

Review articles in *The Obstetrician and Gynaecologist.*

Section 1: General obstetrics

1 Advanced life support

2 Medicolegal issues

GENERAL OBSTETRICS

QUESTIONS

1 Advanced life support

A intravenous adrenaline
B cervical spine stabilisation
C airway securing
D cardiac massage
E intramuscular adrenaline
F assess circulation
G intravenous access and fluids
H chest tube insertion
I resuscitation before laparotomy
J secondary survey
K needle thoracocentesis
L immediate laparoscopy
M assessment of fetal well-being
N burr hole
O chest X-ray
P immediate laparotomy

For each description below, choose the **single** most appropriate answer from the above list of options. Each option may be used once, more than once, or not at all.

1 A 22-year-old pregnant lady is brought to the hospital having been involved in a road traffic accident. She is conscious and communicating verbally, but she becomes increasingly breathless. On examination her pulse is 98 beats/minute and her blood pressure is 100/60 mmHg. Her oxygen saturation is 89 per cent on air. Respiratory examination shows a trachea displaced to the left and asymmetrical chest movements, diminished on the right side. Percussion shows hyperresonance throughout the right side, and breath sounds are muffled on the right.

2 A 22-year-old woman in her fourth pregnancy refers herself to the labour ward following a fall down the stairs. She is 36 weeks pregnant and complaining of abdominal pain. On examination her vital signs demonstrate a pulse of 98 beats/minute and a blood pressure (BP) of 100/60 mmHg. On examination the uterus is tender. On vaginal examination there is no bleeding.

3 A 34-year-old pregnant lady is involved in a road traffic accident. She is 20 weeks into her pregnancy and was a passenger on a motorbike. She is conscious and alert. On examination her pulse is 120 beats/minute and her BP is 90/60 mmHg. She is unable to move her left leg. There is a swelling on her left thigh, with skin bruises.

4 A 24-year-old woman in her first pregnancy presents to Accident and Emergency with acute breathlessness. On examination her lips are swollen. Chest examination reveals an audible wheeze. Her pulse is 110 beats/minute and her BP 100/60 mmHg. Chest examination shows generalised diminished air entry.

Answers: see page 4.

2 Medicolegal issues

A   medical termination of pregnancy
B   inform the parents
C   discuss with a senior colleague
D   seek legal advice
E   take a detailed history
F   inform the police
G   obtain consent and inform the police surgeon
H   surgical termination of pregnancy
I   pregnancy test
J   assess Gillick/Fraser competency
K   inform the General Medical Council
L   inform the police surgeon
M   a person of suitable expertise should conduct an examination
N   offer adoption
O   none of the above

For each description below, choose the **single** most appropriate answer from the above list of options. Each option may be used once, more than once, or not at all.

1   A 12-year-old girl attends the walk-in clinic and requests contraception. Her periods are irregular and her last menstrual period was 6 weeks ago. She has been sexually active for the past 4 months.

2   A 15-year-old girl attends a family planning clinic and requests a termination of pregnancy. Her periods are irregular. An ultrasound scan confirms that she is 8 weeks pregnant. At the consultation she tells you that she does not want her parents to know about her pregnancy or termination.

3   A 23-year-old woman attends Accident and Emergency with vaginal bleeding. On examination she is haemodynamically stable. On vaginal examination there is superficial vaginal trauma and a small tear in the posterior fourchette that requires no intervention. There is extensive bruising to her inner thighs.

Answers: see page 4.

ANSWERS

1 Advanced life support
Answers: H M G A

A 22-year-old pregnant lady is brought to the hospital having been involved in a road traffic accident. She is conscious and communicating verbally, but she becomes increasingly breathless. On examination her pulse is 98 beats/minute and her blood pressure is 100/60 mmHg. Her oxygen saturation is 89 per cent on air. Respiratory examination shows a trachea displaced to the left and asymmetrical chest movements, diminished on the right side. Percussion shows hyperresonance throughout the right side, and breath sounds are muffled on the right.
H   The history is suggestive of a tension pneumothorax.

A 22-year-old woman in her fourth pregnancy refers herself to the labour ward following a fall down the stairs. She is 36 weeks pregnant and complaining of abdominal pain. On examination her vital signs demonstrate a pulse of 98 beats/minute and a blood pressure (BP) of 100/60 mmHg. On examination the uterus is tender. On vaginal examination there is no bleeding.
M   Trauma to the abdomen may predispose to a concealed abruption.

A 34-year-old pregnant lady is involved in a road traffic accident. She is 20 weeks into her pregnancy and was a passenger on a motorbike. She is conscious and alert. On examination her pulse is 120 beats/minute and her BP is 90/60 mmHg. She is unable to move her left leg. There is a swelling on her left thigh, with skin bruises.
G   The picture is suggestive of a long bone fracture. Owing to the large amount of potential blood loss, it is advisable to set up immediate intravenous access.

A 24-year-old woman in her first pregnancy presents to Accident and Emergency with acute breathlessness. On examination her lips are swollen. Chest examination reveals an audible wheeze. Her pulse is 110 beats/minute and her BP 100/60 mmHg. Chest examination shows generalised diminished air entry.
A   Anaphylactic shock needs prompt recognition and administration of adrenaline.

2 Medicolegal issues
Answers: I J E

A 12-year-old girl attends the walk-in clinic and requests contraception. Her periods are irregular and her last menstrual period was 6 weeks ago. She has been sexually active for the past 4 months.
I   Pregnancy needs to be ruled out prior to initiating contraception.

A 15-year-old girl attends a family planning clinic and requests a termination of pregnancy. Her periods are irregular. An ultrasound scan confirms that she is

8 weeks pregnant. At the consultation she tells you that she does not want her parents to know about her pregnancy or termination.

J   A young person under the age of 16 years can give valid consent to a particular intervention or treatment provided he or she fully understands the consequences of the intervention.

A 23-year-old woman attends Accident and Emergency with vaginal bleeding. On examination she is haemodynamically stable. On vaginal examination there is superficial vaginal trauma and a small tear in the posterior fourchette that requires no intervention. There is extensive bruising to her inner thighs.

E   A detailed history is required to establish the cause of trauma before deciding upon the further course of action.

Section 2: Operative obstetrics

3 Caesarean section

4 Obstetric anaesthesia

5 Delivery room management

QUESTIONS

3 Caesarean section

A inform the anaesthetist and senior surgeon, and perform an end-to-end anastomosis
B interrupted non-absorbable sutures and a catheter in situ for 10 days
C caesarean hysterectomy
D inform the anaesthetist and senior surgeon, and perform two-layer closure of the small bowel with absorbable sutures
E single-layer closure
F two-layer closure with absorbable sutures, with a catheter in situ for 2 days
G B Lynch suture
H defunctioning colostomy
I right hemicolectomy
J intramyometrial carboprost
K two-layer closure with non-absorbable sutures and a catheter in situ for 2 days
L interventional radiology and bilateral uterine artery embolisation
M expectant management
N interrupted absorbable sutures and a catheter in situ for 10 days
O unilateral ligation of the uterine artery
P inform the anaesthetist and senior surgeon, and perform two-layer closure of the small bowel with non-absorbable sutures
Q bilateral ligation of the uterine arteries

For each description below, choose the **single** most appropriate answer from the above list of options. Each option may be used once, more than once, or not at all.

1 A 32-year-old lady who is para 2, with a previous caesarean section, undergoes an elective repeat caesarean section. Difficulties are encountered during peritoneal entry. Urine is found to be bloodstained at the end of surgery. A methylene blue test shows a 2 cm rent in the dome of the bladder.

2 A 28-year-old lady undergoes elective surgery for a breech presentation at 39 weeks' gestation. She is known to have undergone bowel surgery as a child. Difficulty is encountered during peritoneal entry. After delivery of the fetus, faecal soiling is noted in the peritoneal cavity. Further exploration reveals a 1 cm size rent in the small bowel.

3 A 26-year-old Jehovah's Witness undergoes a repeat caesarean section for a placenta praevia. Massive postpartum haemorrhage is encountered. The initial medical management and placement of a B Lynch suture are unsuccessful.

Answers: see page 10.

4 Obstetric anaesthesia

A intravenous adrenaline
B caesarean section under spinal anaesthesia
C chest X-ray and antibiotics
D intramuscular adrenaline
E category I caesarean section
F wait and watch
G caesarean section under gas induction
H phenylephrine
I epidural patch
J opioid analgesia
K subcutaneous adrenaline
L check Airway/Breathing/Circulation
M fetal blood sampling
N head-down position
O caesarean section under epidural anaesthesia

For each description below, choose the **single** most appropriate answer from the above list of options. Each option may be used once, more than once, or not at all.

1 A 27-year-old primigravida is being induced at 37 weeks' gestation for pre-eclampsia. Her blood pressure is 140/90 mmHg and she is asymptomatic. Her initial cardiotocograph (CTG) is reactive. She requests pain relief, and an epidural is sited. Her blood pressure falls suddenly to 80/60 mmHg. The CTG shows decelerations with spontaneous recovery. Intravenous fluids are given, and maternal hypotension is persistent with maternal tachycardia of 146 beats/minute.

2 A 36-year-old lady undergoes an elective lower-segment caesarean section (LSCS) for previous LSCS and maternal request. She has an uncomplicated procedure, but on the fourth postoperative day she complains of feeling unwell and being unable to care for her child due to severe headache. Simple analgesics are not helpful.

3 A 27-year-old primigravida is admitted in spontaneous labour at 39 weeks' gestation. She has a prolonged first stage, and fetal decelerations and low pH, for which she undergoes category II caesarean section under spinal anaesthesia. She is complaining of numbness at the level of her nipple and becomes breathless.

4 A 24-year-old primigravida presents in spontaneous labour at term. On vaginal examination a prolapsed pulsating cord is felt. She is rushed to theatre for a category I Caesarean section. Her body mass index is 34, and there is difficulty in intubation.

Answers: see page 10.

5 Delivery room management

A fetal blood sample and forceps delivery in the delivery room
B category I caesarean section
C ventouse delivery in the delivery room
D analgesia
E fetal blood sampling and forceps delivery in theatre
F forceps delivery in theatre
G fetal blood sampling and rotational forceps delivery in theatre
H category II caesarean section
I commence syntocinon
J rotational forceps in the delivery room
K allow a further 30 minutes of active pushing
L rotational forceps in theatre
M none of the above

For each description below, choose the **single** most appropriate answer from the above list of options. Each option may be used once, more than once, or not at all.

1 A 29-year-old woman at term is admitted in spontaneous labour and has progressed to being fully dilated. She has been actively pushing for 60 minutes. On abdominal examination the head is 0/5th palpable. Vaginal examination reveals the position is direct occipitoanterior, there is no caput and moulding, and the station is +2 below the ischial spines.

2 A 29-year-old woman at term is admitted in spontaneous labour and progresses to being fully dilated. The woman has been actively pushing for 60 minutes. On abdominal examination the head is 0/5th palpable. Vaginal examination by the midwife has been unable to determine the position. The station is at the level of the ischial spines.

3 A 29-year-old woman at term is admitted in spontaneous labour and progresses to being fully dilated. She has been actively pushing for 90 minutes. On abdominal examination there is 0/5th of the head palpable. Vaginal examination reveals the position is left occipitotransverse, and there is evidence moulding of 1+ and caput 2+. The station is +1 below the ischial spines.

Answers: see page 11.

ANSWERS

3 Caesarean section

Answers: N D C

A 32-year-old lady who is para 2, with a previous caesarean section, undergoes an elective repeat caesarean section. Difficulties are encountered during peritoneal entry. Urine is found to be bloodstained at the end of surgery. A methylene blue test shows a 2 cm rent in the dome of the bladder.

N   The incidence of bladder damage during caesarean section is about 0.3 per cent. The bladder wall can be repaired by a single continuous or interrupted technique. Postoperatively the catheter needs to be in situ for at least a week.

A 28-year-old lady undergoes elective surgery for a breech presentation at 39 weeks' gestation. She is known to have undergone bowel surgery as a child. Difficulty is encountered during peritoneal entry. After delivery of the fetus, faecal soiling is noted in the peritoneal cavity. Further exploration reveals a 1 cm size rent in the small bowel.

D   Bowel damage is extremely rare during caesarean section and needs full exploration. Small bowel can be repaired in two layers, but large bowel damage requires a temporary defunctioning colostomy.

A 26-year-old Jehovah's Witness undergoes a repeat caesarean section for a placenta praevia. Massive postpartum haemorrhage is encountered. The initial medical management and placement of a B Lynch suture are unsuccessful.

C   In cases of repeat caesarean section with placenta praevia, postpartum haemorrhage should be anticipated and early hysterectomy could be life-saving. Up to 30 per cent of caesarean hysterectomies are done for this indication.

4 Obstetric anaesthesia

Answers: H I L G

A 27-year-old primigravida is being induced at 37 weeks' gestation for pre-eclampsia. Her blood pressure is 140/90 mmHg and she is asymptomatic. Her initial cardiotocograph (CTG) is reactive. She requests pain relief, and an epidural is sited. Her blood pressure falls suddenly to 80/60 mmHg. The CTG shows decelerations with spontaneous recovery. Intravenous fluids are given, and maternal hypotension is persistent with maternal tachycardia of 146 beats/minute.

H   Hypotension following epidural anaesthesia usually settles down with intravenous fluids. If it is persistent, sympathomimetics could be considered by the anaesthetist. Transient hypotension is well tolerated by an otherwise healthy fetus. Persistent fetal distress is an indication for immediate delivery.

A 36-year-old lady undergoes an elective lower-segment caesarean section (LSCS) for previous LSCS and maternal request. She has an uncomplicated procedure, but on the fourth postoperative day she complains of feeling unwell and being unable to care for her child due to severe headache. Simple analgesics are not helpful.

I   Post spinal headache occurs in 2 per cent of cases following epidural anaesthesia and can be managed with a blood patch.

A 27-year-old primigravida is admitted in spontaneous labour at 39 weeks' gestation. She has a prolonged first stage, and fetal decelerations and low pH, for which she undergoes category II caesarean section under spinal anaesthesia. She is complaining of numbness at the level of her nipple and becomes breathless.

L   Checking Airway/Breathing/Circulation is the basic principle in the management of any emergency situation.

A 24-year-old primigravida presents in spontaneous labour at term. On vaginal examination a prolapsed pulsating cord is felt. She is rushed to theatre for a category I caesarean section. Her body mass index is 34, and there is difficulty in intubation.

G   Caesarean section under gas induction is an option for category I Caesarean sections. Obese pregnant women should ideally receive antenatal anaesthetic input.

5 Delivery room management

Answers: C F M

A 29-year-old woman at term is admitted in spontaneous labour and has progressed to being fully dilated. She has been actively pushing for 60 minutes. On abdominal examination the head is 0/5th palpable. Vaginal examination reveals the position is direct occipitoanterior, there is no caput and moulding, and the station is +2 below the ischial spines.

C   Delivery needed at the level of the pelvic outlet can be accomplished with the use of a ventouse cup in the delivery room.

A 29-year-old woman at term is admitted in spontaneous labour and progresses to being fully dilated. The woman has been actively pushing for 60 minutes. On abdominal examination the head is 0/5th palpable. Vaginal examination by the midwife has been unable to determine the position. The station is at the level of the ischial spines.

F   The likely reason for a delay in second stage is malposition of the fetal head. Examination in theatre and delivery by forceps after manual rotation or rotational forceps delivery is appropriate.

A 29-year-old woman at term is admitted in spontaneous labour and progresses to being fully dilated. She has been actively pushing for 90 minutes. On abdominal examination there is 0/5th of the head palpable. Vaginal examination reveals the position is left occipitotransverse, and there is evidence moulding of 1+ and caput 2+. The station is +1 below the ischial spines.

M   A confirmed transverse position of the fetal head with adequate descent into the pelvis may be managed by delivery with rotational forceps in theatre.

Section 3: Medical complications

6 **Breast cancer in pregnancy**

7 **Infections in pregnancy**

8 **Perinatal infection**

9 **HIV infections in pregnancy**

10 **Obstetric cholestasis**

11 **Management of abdominal pain in pregnancy**

12 **Diagnosis of abdominal pain in pregnancy**

13 **Gastrointestinal disorders in pregnancy**

14 **Thromboembolism/venous disorders**

15 **Syncope in pregnancy**

16 **Thyroid diseases complicating pregnancy**

17 **Chest pain in pregnancy**

18 **Diabetes in pregnancy**

19 **Palpitations in pregnancy**

20 **Vomiting/liver function tests in pregnancy**

21 **Medications in pregnancy**

22 **Psychiatric disorders in pregnancy and the puerperium**

23 **Headache**

QUESTIONS

6 Breast cancer in pregnancy

A   ultrasound-guided drainage ± biopsy
B   open surgical drainage
C   radiotherapy with abdominal shielding
D   wide local excision followed by delayed/immediate radiotherapy
E   termination of pregnancy followed by
    surgery + radiotherapy ± chemotherapy
F   radical mastectomy
G   mammogram
H   fine-needle aspiration
I   tamoxifen
J   await spontaneous delivery
K   do nothing
L   defer treatment of cancer until delivery has been induced
M   magnetic resonance imaging
N   ultrasonography ± drainage and antibiotics
O   antibiotics

For each description below, choose the **single** most appropriate answer from the above list of options. Each option may be used once, more than once, or not at all.

1   A 28-year-old lady who is 12 weeks' gestation in her first pregnancy presents to her GP with a painless 2 cm lump in her right breast. She is seen by a specialist surgeon who makes the diagnosis of infiltrative ductal carcinoma on biopsy. The immunohistology of the biopsy demonstrates an oestrogen receptor-positive status.

2   A 39-year-old in her first pregnancy presents at 27 weeks of gestation with a lump in her left breast. Ultrasound examination shows a localised 3 cm lesion in the left breast, and a subsequent biopsy shows a ductal carcinoma.

3   A 29-year-old woman in her first pregnancy is seen at 34 weeks' gestation. She has noticed a lump in her left breast. Further evaluation shows infiltrating duct carcinoma.

4   A primiparous woman presents at 30 weeks' gestation with a painful tender lump in her right breast and fever of 1 week's duration. On examination there is a 4 cm area of induration felt in right breast, with ipsilateral palpable nodes.

Answers: see page 36.

7 Infections in pregnancy

A chloroquine and inpatient care
B oral aciclovir
C neonatal hepatitis B vaccine
D HAART therapy (Highly active anti retroviral therapy)
E interferons/lamivudine
F neonatal observation
G combined active and passive immunisation
H chloroquine prophylaxis
I zoster immunoglobulin and vaccination
J neonatal varicella globulin
K inpatient care and quinine
L neonatal azathioprine therapy
M pyrimethamine and sulphadoxine
N intrapartum antibiotic prophylaxis
O varicella zoster immunoglobulin

For each description below, choose the **single** most appropriate answer from the above list of options. Each option may be used once, more than once, or not at all.

1 A 26-year-old lady attends the antenatal clinic at 18 weeks of gestation following her booking results, which have shown her to be positive for hepatitis B. Antigen analysis demonstrates that she is hepatitis surface antigen positive, hepatitis e antigen negative and anti-Hbe reactive. Her liver function tests are as follows: bilirubin 10 mg/dl, aspartate aminotransferase 36 IU, alanine aminotransferase 40 IU and alkaline phosphatase 600 IU. What is the most appropriate intervention to prevent vertical transmission?

2 A 23-year-old woman in her first pregnancy attends the GP's surgery with a contact history of chickenpox. Her 8-year-old son developed a rash the previous day. She is now 28 weeks pregnant. Her booking bloods show absent exposure/immunity.

3 A 34-year-old woman had a normal vaginal delivery at 36 weeks' gestation. She developed chickenpox on the second postnatal day. The baby is found to be healthy without any obvious lesions. The blood test shows mild thrombocytopenia with a normal haemoglobin level.

4 A 30-year-old woman in her fourth pregnancy is admitted in labour at 37 weeks' gestation. She gives history of sharp radiating pain in the left shoulder and arm with pins and needles. She develops vesicular rashes along the areas of dermatomes C6 and C8 on the second postnatal day.

Answers: see page 36.

8 Perinatal infection

A 10–15 per cent
B 90 per cent
C 50 per cent
D 60–70 per cent
E 80–95 per cent
F 10 per cent
G 20–30 per cent
H 25–40 per cent
I 5 per cent
J <1 per cent
K 100 per cent
L 1–5 per cent
M none of the above

For each description below, choose the **single** most appropriate vertical transmission rate without treatment from the above list of options. Each option may be used once, more than once, or not at all.

1 A 30-year-old woman presents to the clinic at 20 weeks' gestation in her first pregnancy. She is hepatitis B positive. Her serology status is as follows: HBsAg positive, HBeAg positive and hepatitis B virus DNA positive.

2 A 30-year-old woman presents to the clinic at 20 weeks' gestation in her first pregnancy. She is hepatitis C positive. Her serology status is as follows: hepatitis C virus antibody positive, hepatitis virus DNA negative.

3 A 30-year-old woman presents to the clinic at 20 weeks' gestation in her first pregnancy. She is human immunodeficiency virus (HIV) positive.

Answers: see page 37.

9 HIV infections in pregnancy

A   avoid breast-feeding
B   antenatal azathioprine (AZT)
C   antenatal retroviral therapy and elective lower-segment caesarean section (LSCS)
D   inpatient care with intravenous cotrimoxazole and folic acid
E   continuous cardiotocography (CTG)
F   induction at 37 weeks
G   AZT prophylaxis
H   cotrimoxazole and folic acid
I   termination of pregnancy
J   elective LSCS
K   intravenous cotrimoxazole
L   pentamidine
M   emergency LSCS
N   intrapartum AZT and neonatal follow-up
O   HAART (Highly active anti retroviral therapy)
P   antenatal retroviral therapy, elective LSCS and avoidance of breast-feeding
Q   none of the above

For each description below, choose the **single** most appropriate answer from the above list of options. Each option may be used once, more than once, or not at all.

1   A 27-year-old primiparous woman books at 24 weeks' gestation, and her booking bloods show human immunodeficiency (HIV) antibodies, which are later confirmed by polymerase chain reaction. Her CD4 cell count is 1000/mm^3. A fetal anomaly scan is reported as normal. What is the most appropriate option to prevent vertical transmission?

2   A 32-year-old in her first pregnancy, who is known to be HIV positive, is seen in the antenatal clinic at 20 weeks' gestation. Her CD4 cell count is 100/mm^3. What is the most appropriate option?

3   A 20-year-old known intravenous drug abuser presents to Accident and Emergency with a dry cough and breathlessness. She was diagnosed with HIV 2 years ago and has defaulted from further follow-up. She also discloses that she is about 28 weeks pregnant in her first pregnancy. A chest X-ray shows bilateral perihilar interstitial shadows.

Answers: see page 37.

10 Obstetric cholestasis

A   lower-segment caesarean section (LSCS) at term
B   induction at 37 weeks
C   chlorpheniramine
D   elective LSCS at 37 weeks
E   induction at term
F   dexamethasone 10 mg daily for 10 days
G   request serum bile acids
H   S-adenosyl methionine
I   betamethasone administration
J   umbilical artery Doppler scan
K   growth scans
L   emergency caesarean section
M   continuous cardiotocography (CTG)
N   vitamin K
O   urodeoxycholic acid
P   none of the above

For each description below, choose the **single** most appropriate answer from the above list of options. Each option may be used once, more than once, or not at all.

1   A 30-year-old woman in her first pregnancy presents at 30 weeks' gestation with severe itching involving the palms of her hands and soles of her feet. Her liver function tests (LFTs) show normal bilirubin, a mild elevation of serum transaminases and an elevated alkaline phosphatase level. An ultrasound demonstrates normal fetal growth.

2   A 28-year-old woman in her first pregnancy is admitted in labour at 37 weeks' gestation. She has a 5-week history of generalised itching, but on further questioning this is predominately on the soles of her feet and the palms of her hands. LFTs show an elevated alkaline phosphatase, a bilirubin of 20 mg/dl, an aspartate aminotransferase (AST) of 100 IU and an alanine aminotransferase (ALT) of 110 IU. On examination, she is having three contractions every 10 minutes. Vaginal examination reveals that the cervix is 5 cm dilated, and there is meconium-stained liquor.

3   A 27-year-old woman in her first pregnancy attends day assessment unit at 32 weeks' gestation with a history of severe itching and abdominal pain. On abdominal examination the fetal presentation is cephalic and the uterus is noted to be contracting irregularly. Vaginal examination demonstrates that the cervix is 2 cm dilated. Her LFT results are as follows: AST 56 IU, ALT 60 IU, alkaline phosphatase 1000 IU and bilirubin 10 mg/dl. An ultrasound scan demonstrates normal fetal growth and liquor volume. Her autoimmune and viral screens are negative, but bile acids are elevated.

4   A 30-year-old primiparous woman presents at 34 weeks' gestation with severe itching involving the palms of her hands and soles of her feet. LFT shows AST and ALT values of 90 IU and 100 IU respectively. Bile acids are noted to be elevated. A viral screen and autoimmune screen are negative, with normal a coagulation screen. The fetus is appropriately grown for gestation.

Answers: see page 38.

11 Management of abdominal pain in pregnancy

A midstream urine culture and intravenous antibiotic
B conservative management
C cardiotocogram
D appendicectomy
E diagnostic laparoscopy
F laparotomy
G cholecystectomy
H oral antibiotics
I physiotherapy
J stop opioid analgesia
K rehydration with intravenous fluids
L simple analgesia
M laparoscopic removal of cyst/oophorectomy
N bladder catheterisation
O review in 2 weeks
P none of the above

For each description below, choose the **single** most appropriate answer from the above list of options. Each option may be used once, more than once, or not at all.

1 A 22-year-old primiparous woman who is 20 weeks' gestation is admitted with abdominal pain and vomiting. She gives a history of intermittent suprapubic pain that radiates to the flanks. She also describes an increase in urinary frequency, stating that she is passing urine 20 times a day. On examination the uterus is non-tender; however, there is a degree of suprapubic tenderness with bilateral flank tenderness. The maternal temperature is noted to be 38.6°C. Urine analysis shows a white cell count of 100/mm^3.

2 A 34-year-old Afro-Caribbean lady is admitted to the delivery suite at 32 weeks' gestation with severe abdominal pain. She is a known sickle cell disease patient. Ultrasound shows a normally grown fetus with no obvious uterine fibroids. She had an episode of diarrhoea 3 days ago. Abdominal and vaginal examination are normal.

3 A 25-year-old woman who is 36 weeks' gestation in her first pregnancy is on the ward because she has symphysis pubis dysfunction. She is taking paracetamol and codeine phosphate for the pain. She has not opened her bowels since admission. She now has generalised abdominal pain that is not aggravated or relieved by anything. On examination her abdomen is generally tender all over. The uterus is soft, and fetal movements are felt.

4 A 32-year-old primiparous woman presents at 20 weeks' gestation with a sudden onset of severe epigastric pain radiating to her back. She has recently noticed epigastric and right hypochondrial discomfort with fatty meals. Blood results are all normal except for an amylase of 1600 IU. Ultrasound shows multiple gallstones with a normal common bile duct. The pancreas and liver appear normal.

Answers: see page 39.

12 Diagnosis of abdominal pain in pregnancy

A mesenteric vein thrombosis

B pancreatitis

C appendicitis

D ureteric colic

E pyelonephritis

F torsion of an ovarian cyst

G pre-eclampsia

H red degeneration

I HELLP (*h*aemolytic anaemia, *e*levated *l*iver enzymes and *l*ow *p*latelet count) syndrome

J acute fatty liver

K severe constipation

L abruption

M preterm labour

N urinary retention

O sickle cell crisis

P Crohn's disease

Q ulcerative colitis

R none of the above

For each description below, choose the **single** most appropriate answer from the above list of options. Each option may be used once, more than once, or not at all.

1 An 18-year-old primigravida is admitted with severe abdominal pain at 28 weeks' gestation. She describes the pain to be radiating from her back to her groin. She was treated for an episode of fever with chills a month ago by her GP. Urinalysis showed leucocytes and blood. Her blood test results are as follows: haemoglobin 10.7 g/dL, white blood cell count 17×10^9/L platelets 187×10^9/L, uric acid 0.30 mmol/L, amylase 250 u/dL, aspartate aminotransferase (AST) 17 IU/L and alanine aminotransferase 23 IU/L.

2 A 35-year-old lady attends the day assessment unit with abdominal pain. She is 32 weeks pregnant in her fourth pregnancy. She also gives a history of nausea and vomiting since the morning. There is no history of tightening, or bleeding per vaginum. She drinks 20 units of alcohol a week. Her blood pressure is 130/86 mmHg and her pulse 100 beats/minute. Urine analysis is negative. Her blood results are: haemoglobin 13.7 gm/dl, white blood cell count 14×10^9/L, C-reactive protein (CRP) 200 units, AST 40 IU, gamma-glutamyl transferase (GGT) 50 IU, alkaline phosphatase (ALP) 200 IU, amylase 900 IU and bilirubin 28 mmol/L.

3 A 24-year-old primigravida presents to Accident and Emergency at 32 weeks' gestation with a history of acute abdominal pain. She is agitated and confused, and she also has headache and severe nausea. There is no history of tightenings or bleeding per vaginum. Her blood pressure is 130/86 mmHg and urinalysis

shows 3+ protein. Her initial blood results are: haemoglobin 11.7 gm/dl, white blood cell count 9.0 cells/mm^3, CRP 100 units, AST 100 IU, GGT 97 IU, ALP 600 IU, bilirubin 22 mg/dl, amylase 60 IU and serum albumin 25 g/dl.

4 A 28-year-old primigravida presents with lower abdominal pain at 14 weeks' gestation. There is no history of vaginal bleeding or dysuria. She has had an episode of vomiting in the morning. On examination her temperature is 37.8°C. There is tenderness in her lower abdomen, particularly the right lower quadrant. Vaginal examination reveals a closed cervix with no bleeding. Blood results are: haemoglobin 11.7 gm/dl, white blood cell count 17.0 cells/mm^3, CRP 100 units, AST 30 IU, GGT 17 IU, ALP 150 IU, bilirubin 22 mg/dl, amylase 50 IU and serum albumin 25 g/dl.

Answers: see page 40.

13 Gastrointestinal disorders in pregnancy

A   stool softeners
B   drainage of thrombosed haemorrhoid
C   ice pack and analgesics
D   haemorrhoidectomy
E   oral steroids
F   corticosteroid/mesalazine enema
G   infliximab (a tumour necrosis factor inhibitor)
H   drainage of sepsis ± setons
I   fistulectomy
J   arachis oil enema
K   do nothing
L   sclerosant
M   lateral anal sphincterotomy
N   defunctioning colostomy
O   maximal anal dilatation
P   none of the above

For each description below, choose the **single** most appropriate answer from the above list of options. Each option may be used once, more than once, or not at all.

1   A 30-year-old woman who has a longstanding history of Crohn's disease is admitted at 28 weeks' gestation in her first pregnancy with multiple fistulae around the anus, which are associated with abscess formation.

2   A 32-year-old pregnant woman presents with a painful perianal lump of 4 days' duration in the third trimester. She is known to have had problems with haemorrhoids in the past. On examination there are tender prolapsed circumferential haemorrhoids.

3   A 34-year-old pregnant lady presents at 30 weeks' gestation with severe tenesmus and intermittent bleeding per rectum. Rigid sigmoidoscopy shows an inflamed rectum. Rectal biopsies have been reported to be suggestive of ulcerative colitis.

Answers: see page 41.

14 Thromboembolism/venous disorders

A   injection sclerotherapy
B   bilateral saphenofemoral ligation and multiple stab avulsion under local anaesthesia
C   bilateral saphenofemoral ligation under general anaesthesia
D   compression stockings and leg elevation
E   embolectomy
F   stripping of the long saphenous vein
G   intravenous heparin 10 000 units bolus followed by full heparinisation
H   enoxaparin 40 mg once daily
I   warfarin with an international normalised ratio of 3–4
J   bed rest
K   heparin 10 000 units twice daily
L   stop warfarin and switch to heparin
M   perform a thrombophilia screen until the activated partial thromboplastin time is 1.5–2 times the reference value
N   enoxaparin 1.5 mg/kg per day

For each description below, choose the **single** most appropriate answer from the above list of options. Each option may be used once, more than once, or not at all.

1   A 31-year-old woman presents at 34 weeks' gestation with a dull ache in her left calf. She is a smoker, and on examination there are superficial varicose veins present on both sides with localised left calf tenderness. Doppler studies show a loss of patency of the left long saphenous vein with a thrombus extending for 5 cm along the left popliteal fossa.

2   A 31-year-old woman presents at 34 weeks' gestation with severe pain in both calves. The pain generally worsens over the day. On examination there are marked varicosities involving the long saphenous territory. Duplex examination shows bilateral saphenofemoral reflux. Doppler studies confirm normal patency of the deep venous system of both legs.

3   A 31-year-old woman presents at 34 weeks' gestation with a twin pregnancy with pain in her right calf. She is a smoker and her body mass index is 34 at booking. On examination she has bilateral varicose veins and right-sided superficial thrombophlebitis. Doppler studies report normal patency of the deep venous system of both legs. She has a family history of antithrombin III deficiency.

Answers: see page 41.

15 Syncope in pregnancy

A supine hypotension
B thyrotoxicosis
C arrhythmias
D aortic stenosis
E postural hypotension
F labyrinthitis
G Menière's disease
H anaemia
I hypertrophic obstructive cardiomyopathy
J vasovagal attack
K electrolyte imbalance
L hypoglycaemia
M intracranial mass
N cervical spondylosis
O meningitis
P none of the above

For each description below, choose the **single** most appropriate answer from the above list of options. Each option may be used once, more than once, or not at all.

1 A 30-year-old primigravid woman presents at 12 weeks' gestation. She is complaining of dizziness and vertigo. She states that she had a chest infection a week ago. On examination her dizziness is worse on turning her head. Her pulse and blood pressure are normal. She also has demonstrable nystagmus.

2 A 30-year-old lady who is in her second pregnancy attends the antenatal clinic for her booking. She complains of feeling dizzy after her booking blood tests. She has no prior history of dizziness. On examination her pulse rate is found to be 45 beats/minute, and her blood pressure is 120/76 mmHg. She has no neurological signs.

3 A 30-year-old lady presents in her second pregnancy at 34 weeks' gestation with dizziness. She is otherwise well with no other medical problems. She states that her dizziness is worse in the mornings and is relieved by rest. On examination her vital signs are normal. A full blood count demonstrates that her haemoglobin is 13.1 g/dL.

Answers: see page 42.

16 Thyroid diseases complicating pregnancy

A total thyroidectomy
B hemithyroidectomy
C watchful expectancy
D beta-blockers and supportive measures
E propylthiouracil
F thyroxine
G block and replacement regimens
H chlorambucil
I supportive measures
J steroid administration
K anti-arrhythmic drugs
L amiodarone
M thiopentone
N radioactive iodine
O propylthiouracil and thyroxine

For each description below, choose the **single** most appropriate answer from the above list of options. Each option may be used once, more than once, or not at all.

1 A 34-year-old primigravida is admitted to the antenatal ward. She is 18 weeks pregnant. She complains of a 2-day history of vomiting and a feeling that her heart has been beating faster on several occasions. On examination she looks anxious. She has a persistent pulse rate of 110 beats/minute and blood pressure of 140/70 mmHg. On examination of the hands she has a fine tremor. Thyroid function tests (TFTs) show a free thyroxine (T4) of 200 nmol/L (normal range 70–140 nmol/L), a tri-iodothyronine (T3) of 6 nmol/L (1.2–3.0 nmol/L) and a thyroid-stimulating hormone (TSH) level of 0.1 μ/L (0.5–5.0 nmol/L). The electrocardiograph shows sinus tachycardia.

2 A 27-year-old lady presents 12 weeks after the birth of her first child. She is complaining of a painful swelling in her neck and her heart beating faster. On examination her pulse is 110 beats/minute. Her thyroid gland is enlarged and non-tender. Her TFTs show a free T4 of 180 nmol/L (70–140 nmol/L), a T3 of 8 nmol/L (1.2–3.0 nmol/L) and a TSH of 0.28 μ/L (0.5–5.0 nmol/L). Radioactive iodine uptake shows a low uptake into the thyroid gland.

3 A 27-year-old woman presents at 24 weeks' gestation in her first pregnancy. She complains of a swelling in her neck. On examination the thyroid gland is enlarged and tender. She states that she had a sore throat and generalized malaise 2 weeks ago. Her TFTs show a free T4 of 160 nmol/L (70–140 nmol/L), a T3 of 6 nmol/L (1.2–3.0 nmol/L) and a TSH of 0.1 μ/L (0.5–5.0 nmol/L).

4 A 27-year-old woman is referred to antenatal clinic at 28 weeks' gestation in her first pregnancy. The community midwife has measured the symphysis–fundus

height at 24 cm. The woman is known to be hypothyroid secondarily to Graves' disease and is currently taking thyroxine supplementation. On examination the symphysis–fundus height measures 25 cm. The woman's TFTs show a free T4 of 86 nmol/L (70–140 nmol/L), a T3 of 2.1 (1.2–3.0 nmol/L) and a TSH of 2.2 μ/L (0.5–5.0 nmol/L) level. Ultrasound demonstrates a fetal goitre with fetal heart rate of 200 beats/minute. Abdominal circumference and head circumference are on the third centile. Umbilical artery Doppler studies are normal.

Answers: see page 42.

17 Chest pain in pregnancy

A   tuberculous cavitation

B   pulmonary embolism

C   musculoskeletal pain

D   gastro-oesophageal reflux

E   pneumonia

F   pneumothorax

G   ischaemic heart disease

H   aortic stenosis

I   cardiac tamponade

J   myocarditis

K   aortic dissection

L   pleural effusion

M   anaemia

N   pericardial effusion

O   costochondritis

P   none of the above

For each description below, choose the **single** most appropriate answer from the above list of options. Each option may be used once, more than once, or not at all.

1   A 46-year-old lady who conceived with ovum donation presents at 34 weeks' gestation with a sudden onset of central chest pain and breathlessness. She smokes about 15 cigarettes a day. On examination, her pulse is 98 beats/minute and her blood pressure (BP) is 100/70 mmHg. The symphysis–fundus height is appropriate for gestation, and the fetal heart is heard normally. The chest X-ray is reported to be normal. An electrocardiogram (ECG) shows a sinus rhythm with T wave inversion noted in leads III, aVL and aVF.

2   A 26-year-old woman presents at 27 weeks' gestation in her second pregnancy with severe chest pain that radiates to her back. Her height is 170 cm and she has been noted to have hypermobile joints. On examination she looks unwell with a pulse rate of 136 beats/minute and a BP of 76/46 mmHg. The chest X-ray is reported to be normal. An ECG shows sinus rhythm with a rate of 128 beats/minute.

3   A 32-year-old Asian lady who has recently moved to the UK presents at 20 weeks' gestation in her third pregnancy with left-sided chest pain. She describes becoming increasingly breathless over the past 4 weeks. She gives a recent history of easy fatigability and lassitude. On examination her pulse rate is 88 beats/minute and her BP is 96/70 mmHg. Auscultation of the heart reveals muffled heart sounds. An ECG shows low-voltage complexes.

4   A 30-year-old schoolteacher presents at 30 weeks' gestation with right-sided chest pain, which is made worse on coughing. She also complains of a productive cough. On examination her pulse is 110 beats/minute and her BP is 100/76 mmHg. Her temperature is 38°C. The heart sounds are normal, and breath sounds are diminished on the right side. The chest X-ray shows a ground-glass appearance on the right side.

Answers: see page 43.

18 Diabetes in pregnancy

A   insulin administration
B   decrease the insulin dose
C   dietary advice
D   glycosylated haemoglobin
E   induction at 37 weeks
F   elective lower-segment caesarean section at term
G   increase the insulin dose
H   glucose tolerance test (GTT)
I   watchful expectancy
J   anticipate shoulder dystocia
K   fasting blood sugar
L   random blood glucose
M   induction at 38 weeks
N   induction at term
O   none of the above

For each description below, choose the **single** most appropriate answer from the above list of options. Each option may be used once, more than once, or not at all.

1   A 27-year-old lady is 26 weeks pregnant in her second pregnancy. In her first pregnancy she had an emergency caesarean section for failure to progress. The baby weighed 4.0 kg. She has an oral glucose tolerance test and her results are as follows: fasting glucose 7.2 mmol/L, 2-hour postprandial glucose 10.8 mmol/L.

2   A known insulin-dependent diabetic patient attends the combined clinic for follow-up and is found to have inadequately controlled glycaemia with an increasing glucose level.

3   A woman with diet-controlled gestational diabetes mellitus is seen in the antenatal clinic at 33 weeks' gestation and found to have a symphysis–fundus height of 37 cm. Her blood sugar values over the last 2 weeks have been progressively increasing in spite of good dietary restrictions.

4   A 30-year-old lady who had a stillbirth in her previous pregnancy has been found to have undiagnosed diabetes. She is currently on oral hypoglycaemic agents, with good glycaemic control, and attends for prepregnancy counselling. What is the appropriate next step?

Answers: see page 44.

19 Palpitations in pregnancy

A   physiological
B   phaeochromocytoma
C   ventricular ectopic beats
D   sinus tachycardia
E   anaemia
F   supraventricular tachycardia
G   atrial fibrillation
H   heart block
I   re-entry tachycardia
J   junctional rhythm
K   thyrotoxicosis
L   Wolff–Parkinson–White syndrome
M   mitral valve prolapse
N   myocarditis
O   anxiety neurosis
P   none of the above

For each description below, choose the **single** most appropriate answer from the above list of options. Each option may be used once, more than once, or not at all.

1   A 35-year-old lady who is para 2 presents with palpitations. She has associated non-proteinuric hypertension inadequately controlled by methyldopa. She is complaining of intermittent headaches and sweating.

2   A 27-year-old anxious-looking primigravid woman presents at 18 weeks' gestation with palpitations and tremors. Her haemoglobin level is 112 mg/dl. An electrocardiogram shows sinus tachycardia.

3   A 32-year-old lady of oriental origin presents at 18 weeks' gestation with palpitations. She has a long history of breathlessness. She also recollects having swollen joints and fever in childhood.

4   A healthy pregnant woman attends for her booking at 34 weeks' gestation. She mentions occasional palpitations with no other associated symptoms. Her haemoglobin is 12.1 g/dL.

Answers: see page 45.

20 Vomiting/liver function tests in pregnancy

A HELLP (*h*aemolytic anaemia, *e*levated *l*iver enzymes and *l*ow *p*latelets) syndrome

B viral hepatitis

C obstetric cholestasis

D acute fatty liver of pregnancy

E chronic active hepatitis

F hyperemesis gravidarum

G physiological changes

H primary biliary cirrhosis

I autoimmune hepatitis

J sclerosing cholangitis

K severe pre-eclampsia

L drug-induced hepatitis

M pancreatitis

N gallstones

O lichen sclerosis

For each description below, choose the **single** most appropriate answer from the above list of options. Each option may be used once, more than once, or not at all.

1 A 23-year-old primigravida presents at 36 weeks' gestation with severe generalised itching and sleeplessness. Liver function tests (LFTs) are as follows: bilirubin 10 mg/dl, aspartate aminotransferase (AST) 35 IU, alanine aminotransferase (ALT) 40 IU and alkaline phosphatase 1000 IU. What is the most likely diagnosis?

2 A 28-year-old lady who is para 2 presents at 12 weeks' gestation with fever, malaise and vomiting. LFTs arranged by her GP are as follows: bilirubin 24 mg/dl, AST 100 IU, ALT 120 IU and alkaline phosphatase 800 IU. What is the most likely diagnosis?

3 A 32-year-old primipara presents at 32 weeks' gestation with severe itching involving her palms and soles. LFTs are as follows: bilirubin 10 mg/dl, AST 50 IU, ALT 58 IU, alkaline phosphatase 660 IU and bile acids 26 mg/dl. What is the most likely diagnosis?

4 A 19-year-old girl presents at 32 weeks' gestation with nausea, vomiting, abdominal pain and severe malaise of 2 days' duration. On examination her Glasgow coma score is 11. She was diagnosed with mild pre-eclampsia at 28 weeks' gestation. LFTs show bilirubin 24 mg/dl, AST 100 IU and ALT 120 IU. What is the most likely diagnosis?

5 A 25-year-old woman presents at 18 weeks' gestation with severe blood-stained vomiting and tiredness. On examination she is dehydrated. LFTs are as

follows: bilirubin 10 mg/dl, AST 50 IU, ALT 45 IU, alkaline phosphatase 480 IU. Her haematocrit is 0.48 l/L, and urine analysis shows ketones. What is the most likely diagnosis?

6   A 24-year-old pregnant lady presents at 20 weeks' gestation with severe abdominal pain and dehydration. She has recently been diagnosed with gallstones. LFTs are as follows: bilirubin 25 mg/dl, amylase 1000 IU, AST 60 IU, ALT 68 IU and alkaline phosphatase 1500 IU. What is the most likely diagnosis?

Answers: see page 45.

21 Medications in pregnancy

A   calcium supplements
B   erythromycin
C   nifedipine
D   ritodrine
E   ursodeoxycholic acid
F   atosiban
G   sodium valproate
H   labetalol
I   carbamazepine
J   ramipril
K   methyldopa
L   aspirin 75 mg
M   sodium nitroprusside
N   phenytoin
O   lamotrigine
P   atenolol
Q   none of the above

For each description below, choose the **single** most appropriate drug from the above list of options. Each option may be used once, more than once, or not at all.

1   A 32-week primigravid lady is admitted to the labour ward with irregular tightenings. She denies any history of bleeding per vaginum or draining. She is an ex-smoker who recently quit smoking. There are no significant medical or surgical problems. On examination the presentation is cephalic and the cervix is posterior and closed. Urine analysis is negative. The woman is then given the stat dose of a tocolytic, after which she develops a severe headache, hypotension and flushing.

2   A 38-year-old primigravida is currently 22 weeks pregnant and is being seen in the antenatal clinic following her anomaly scan. She is known to have epilepsy, for which she is on medication. The initial scan was incomplete as the facial anatomy was difficult to achieve. A subsequent detailed scan confirms a cleft lip. The woman's last episode of fits was a year ago.

3   A 22-year-old lady is admitted to the labour ward at 34 weeks' gestation. She was diagnosed with pre-eclampsia and was started on medication 2 weeks ago. She is feeling low and depressed but denies any history of headache or visual disturbances. On examination her reflexes are normal and there is an adequately grown fetus. Her blood pressure is 130/76 mmHg and there is 1+ proteinuria. Her renal function and liver function tests are normal.

Answers: see page 46.

22 Psychiatric disorders in pregnancy and the puerperium

A baby blues
B postnatal depression
C panic disorders
D schizophrenia
E puerperal psychosis
F bipolar affective disorder
G depression
H withdrawal psychosis
I personality disorder
J space-occupying lesions
K acute confusional state
L metabolic disorder
M post-traumatic stress disorder
N none of the above

For each description below, choose the **single** most appropriate answer from the above list of options. Each option may be used once, more than once, or not at all.

1   A 23-year-old woman who has had a normal delivery 12 hours earlier is noted by the ward staff to be having difficulties sleeping, is overactive and expresses feelings of excitement.

2   A 23-year-old woman presents at the booking clinic. She is 7 weeks pregnant in her first pregnancy and has been referred by the community midwife for consultant care. She feels well in herself and says that a specific voice has been speaking to her every morning instructing her to do things. She is not on any medication.

3   A 40-year-old woman presents on the fifth day after a normal delivery. Her husband brought her in to Accident and Emergency after he noticed an abrupt change in her behaviour. He describes her as confused, restless and expressing thoughts of self-harm.

Answers: see page 47.

23 Headache

A   aseptic meningitis
B   bacterial meningitis
C   brain abscess
D   brain metastases
E   cerebrovascular occlusion
F   cluster headache
G   hypertensive crisis
H   infective endocarditis
I   migraine
J   primary brain tumour
K   tension headache
L   subarachnoid haemorrhage
M   trigeminal neuralgia
N   benign intracranial hypertension
O   pre-eclampsia
P   iatrogenic headache
Q   none of the above

For each description below, choose the **single** most appropriate diagnosis from the answers in the above list of options. Each option may be used once, more than once, or not at all.

1   A 32-year-old lady is admitted via the Accident and Emergency unit with sudden severe unilateral right-sided headache at 12 weeks' gestation. She is noted to have swelling around her right eye. Her blood pressure is normal and there are no focal neurological signs. There is no history of migraines.

2   A 38-year-old lady presents to the labour ward with headache. She works as a manager and is currently 24 weeks pregnant. She describes it as a squeezing type of pain in her forehead. Her blood pressure and neurological examination are normal.

3   A 39-year-old lady attends the day unit with headache. She is 26 weeks' pregnant and was on captopril, which was later converted to methyldopa at booking. Nifedipine has recently been added to her medication. There is no proteinuria and she denies any history of visual disturbances. On examination her reflexes are normal.

4   A 23-year-old primigravida is seen in the day unit for severe headache of insidious origin and associated vomiting without any nausea. She is 28 weeks pregnant in her second pregnancy and has no proteinuria. Her blood pressure is 90/60 mmHg and her pulse rate 78 beats/minute. There is no significant medical or surgical history. Initial blood investigations are normal. Fundoscopy reveals bilateral papilloedema.

Answers: see page 47.

ANSWERS

6 Breast cancer in pregnancy

Answers: E D L N

A 28-year-old lady who is 12 weeks' gestation in her first pregnancy presents to her GP with a painless 2 cm lump in her right breast. She is seen by a specialist surgeon who makes the diagnosis of infiltrative ductal carcinoma on biopsy. The immunohistology of the biopsy demonstrates an oestrogen receptor-positive status.

E   With the finding of an infiltrative ductal carcinoma there is a significant chance that the patient will require some form of adjuvant therapy after surgery. Therefore if chemotherapy is required in the first trimester of pregnancy, termination of pregnancy should be proposed owing to the possible teratogenic effects. If, however, the patient wishes to continue with the pregnancy, adjuvant therapy should be delayed until the second trimester.

A 39- year-old in her first pregnancy presents at 27 weeks of gestation with a lump in her left breast. Ultrasound examination shows a localised 3 cm lesion in the left breast, and a subsequent biopsy shows a ductal carcinoma.

D   For early-stage cancer detected in the second trimester, lumpectomy can be followed by chemotherapy, and radiation can be withheld until after birth.

A 29-year-old woman in her first pregnancy is seen at 34 weeks' gestation. She has noticed a lump in her left breast. Further evaluation shows infiltrating duct carcinoma.

L   If an invasive cancer is detected close to term, treatment can be deferred for a short period until after delivery.

A primiparous woman presents at 30 weeks' gestation with a painful tender lump in her right breast and fever of 1 week's duration. On examination there is a 4 cm area of induration felt in right breast, with ipsilateral palpable nodes.

N   Ultrasound is useful for guided aspiration and to exclude residual lumps as inflammatory breast cancer can present as breast abscess.

7 Infections in pregnancy

Answers: C O J F

A 26-year-old lady attends the antenatal clinic at 18 weeks of gestation following her booking results, which have shown her to be positive for hepatitis B. Antigen analysis demonstrates that she is hepatitis surface antigen positive, hepatitis e antigen negative and anti-Hbe reactive. Her liver function tests are as follows: bilirubin 10 mg/dl, aspartate aminotransferase 36 IU, alanine aminotransferase 40 IU and alkaline phosphatase 600 IU. What is the most appropriate intervention to prevent vertical transmission?

C   Neonatal active immunisation is indicated in babies born to mothers with low infectivity as suggested by e antigen negativity.

A 23-year-old woman in her first pregnancy attends the GP's surgery with a contact history of chickenpox. Her 8-year-old son developed a rash the previous day. She is now 28 weeks pregnant. Her booking bloods show absent exposure/immunity.
O   Varicella zoster immunoglobulin can be given with a history of contact with chickenpox from 24 hours up to 10 days.

A 34-year-old woman had a normal vaginal delivery at 36 weeks' gestation. She developed chickenpox on the second postnatal day. The baby is found to be healthy without any obvious lesions. The blood test shows mild thrombocytopenia with a normal haemoglobin level.
J   Neonatal zoster immunoglobulin can be given if maternal infection occurs 5 days before and 2 days after delivery.

A 30-year-old woman in her fourth pregnancy is admitted in labour at 37 weeks' gestation. She gives history of sharp radiating pain in the left shoulder and arm with pins and needles. She develops vesicular rashes along the areas of dermatomes C6 and C8 on the second postnatal day.
F   Maternal shingles does not pose a risk to the fetus or the neonate as the baby is protected by passively acquired maternal immunity.

8 Perinatal infection

Answers: E J G

A 30-year-old woman presents to the clinic at 20 weeks' gestation in her first pregnancy. She is hepatitis B positive. Her serology status is as follows: HBsAg positive, HBeAg positive and hepatitis B virus DNA positive.
E   A serum positive status for hepatitis B e antigen and the presence of viral DNA is associated with a very high risk of perinatal transmission.

A 30-year-old woman presents to the clinic at 20 weeks' gestation in her first pregnancy. She is hepatitis C positive. Her serology status is as follows: hepatitis C virus antibody positive, hepatitis virus DNA negative.
J   Hepatitis C infection with absent serum DNA confers a low risk of perinatal infection.

A 30-year-old woman presents to the clinic at 20 weeks' gestation in her first pregnancy. She is human immunodeficiency virus (HIV) positive.
G   HIV-positive status without any treatment or medical intervention confers a risk of perinatal transmission of 20–30 per cent.

9 HIV infections in pregnancy

Answers: P H D

A 27-year-old primiparous woman books at 24 weeks' gestation, and her booking bloods show human immunodeficiency (HIV) antibodies, which are later

confirmed by polymerase chain reaction. Her CD4 cell count is 1000/mm^3. A fetal anomaly scan is reported as normal. What is the most appropriate option to prevent vertical transmission?

P   These interventions are shown to reduce the risk of vertical transmission from 30 per cent to 2 per cent.

A 32-year-old in her first pregnancy, who is known to be HIV positive, is seen in the antenatal clinic at 20 weeks' gestation. Her CD4 cell count is 100/mm^3. What is the most appropriate option?

H   *Pneumocystis carinii* pneumonia prophylaxis needs to be started with cotrimoxazole and folic acid when the CD4 cell count falls below 200 cells/mm^3.

A 20-year-old known intravenous drug abuser presents to Accident and Emergency with a dry cough and breathlessness. She was diagnosed with HIV 2 years ago and has defaulted from further follow-up. She also discloses that she is about 28 weeks pregnant in her first pregnancy. A chest X-ray shows bilateral perihilar interstitial shadows.

D   Inpatient care is needed for patients with pneumonia.

10 Obstetric cholestasis

Answers: G M I N

A 30-year-old woman in her first pregnancy presents at 30 weeks' gestation with severe itching involving the palms of her hands and soles of her feet. Her liver function tests (LFTs) show normal bilirubin, a mild elevation of serum transaminases and an elevated alkaline phosphatase level. An ultrasound demonstrates normal fetal growth.

G   Elevated bile acids establish the diagnosis of obstetric cholestasis.

A 28-year-old woman in her first pregnancy is admitted in labour at 37 weeks' gestation. She has a 5-week history of generalised itching, but on further questioning this is predominately on the soles of her feet and the palms of her hands. LFTs show an elevated alkaline phosphatase, a bilirubin of 20 mg/dl, an aspartate aminotransferase (AST) of 100 IU and an alanine aminotransferase (ALT) of 110 IU. On examination, she is having three contractions every 10 minutes. Vaginal examination reveals that the cervix is 5 cm dilated, and there is meconium-stained liquor.

M   Obstetric cholestasis is an indication for continuous CTG in labour.

A 27-year-old woman in her first pregnancy attends day assessment unit at 32 weeks' gestation with a history of severe itching and abdominal pain. On abdominal examination the fetal presentation is cephalic and the uterus is noted to be contracting irregularly. Vaginal examination demonstrates that the cervix is 2 cm dilated. Her LFT results are as follows: AST 56 IU, ALT 60 IU, alkaline phosphatase 1000 IU and bilirubin 10 mg/dl. An ultrasound scan demonstrates normal fetal growth and liquor volume. Her autoimmune and viral screens are negative, but bile acids are elevated.

I   Preterm labour is common in obstetric cholestasis, and steroids are indicated up to 34 weeks' gestation.

A 30-year-old primiparous woman presents at 34 weeks' gestation with severe itching involving the palms of her hands and soles of her feet. LFT shows AST and ALT values of 90 IU and 100 IU respectively. Bile acids are noted to be elevated. A viral screen and autoimmune screen are negative, with normal a coagulation screen. The fetus is appropriately grown for gestation.

N   Although obstetric cholestasis is widely regarded by obstetricians to be an indication for induction of labour at term, there is little evidence to support this practice. The recent Royal College of Obstetricians and Gynaecologists' (RCOG) guideline suggests that early induction should be on an individual basis after consideration of the possible neonatal consequences. The RCOG also suggest that there is insufficient evidence to support treatment regimens outside research trials. However, it does suggest that it is reasonable to offer vitamin K.

11 Management of abdominal pain in pregnancy

Answers: A K J G

A 22-year-old primiparous woman who is 20 weeks' gestation is admitted with abdominal pain and vomiting. She gives a history of intermittent suprapubic pain that radiates to the flanks. She also describes an increase in urinary frequency, stating that she is passing urine 20 times a day. On examination the uterus is non-tender; however, there is a degree of suprapubic tenderness with bilateral flank tenderness. The maternal temperature is noted to be 38.6°C. Urine analysis shows a white cell count of 100/mm³.

A   Pyelonephritis needs appropriate antibiotic treatment in pregnancy.

A 34-year-old Afro-Caribbean lady is admitted to the delivery suite at 32 weeks' gestation with severe abdominal pain. She is a known sickle cell disease patient. Ultrasound shows a normally grown fetus with no obvious uterine fibroids. She had an episode of diarrhoea 3 days ago. Abdominal and vaginal examination are normal.

K   Sickle cell crisis could be precipitated by dehydration and needs aggressive fluid therapy.

A 25-year-old woman who is 36 weeks' gestation in her first pregnancy is on the ward because she has symphysis pubis dysfunction. She is taking paracetamol and codeine phosphate for the pain. She has not opened her bowels since admission. She now has generalised abdominal pain that is not aggravated or relieved by anything. On examination her abdomen is generally tender all over. The uterus is soft, and fetal movements are felt.

J   Opiates are considered to be good analgesics in pregnancy but could result in severe constipation.

A 32-year-old primiparous woman presents at 20 weeks' gestation with a sudden onset of severe epigastric pain radiating to her back. She has recently noticed

epigastric and right hypochondrial discomfort with fatty meals. Blood results are all normal except for an amylase of 1600 IU. Ultrasound shows multiple gallstones with a normal common bile duct. The pancreas and liver appear normal.

G   Laparoscopic cholecystectomy can be safely performed during pregnancy if indicated.

12 Diagnosis of abdominal pain in pregnancy

Answers: E B J C

An 18-year-old primigravida is admitted with severe abdominal pain at 28 weeks' gestation. She describes the pain to be radiating from her back to her groin. She was treated for an episode of fever with chills a month ago by her GP. Urinalysis showed leucocytes and blood. Her blood test results are as follows: haemoglobin 10.7 gm/dl, white blood cell count 17.0 cells/mm^3 platelets 187 cells/mm^3, uric acid 0.30 gm/dl, amylase 250 IU, aspartate aminotransferase (AST) 17 IU and alanine aminotransferase 23 IU.

E   Pyelonephritis is common in pregnancy due to physiological changes in the urinary tract during pregnancy.

A 35-year-old lady attends the day assessment unit with abdominal pain. She is 32 weeks pregnant in her fourth pregnancy. She also gives a history of nausea and vomiting since the morning. There is no history of tightening, or bleeding per vaginum. She drinks 20 units of alcohol a week. Her blood pressure is 130/86 mmHg and her pulse 100 beats/minute. Urine analysis is negative. Her blood results are: haemoglobin 13.7 gm/dl, white blood cell count 14.0 cells/mm^3, C-reactive protein (CRP) 200 units, AST 40 IU, gamma-glutamyl transferase (GGT) 50 IU, alkaline phosphatase (ALP) 200 IU, amylase 900 IU and bilirubin 28 mg/dl.

B   Gallstones and alcoholism are the common causes of acute pancreatitis, and treatment is intensive supportive therapy.

A 24-year-old primigravida presents to Accident and Emergency at 32 weeks' gestation with a history of acute abdominal pain. She is agitated and confused, and she also has headache and severe nausea. There is no history of tightenings or bleeding per vaginum. Her blood pressure is 130/86 mmHg and urinalysis shows 3+ protein. Her initial blood results are: haemoglobin 11.7 gm/dl, white blood cell count 9.0 cells/mm^3, CRP 100 units, AST 100 IU, GGT 97 IU, ALP 600 IU, bilirubin 22 mg/dl, amylase 60 IU and serum albumin 25 g/dl.

J   Acute fatty liver is rare in pregnancy but the prognosis is poor. It usually occurs in patients with pre-eclampsia.

A 28-year-old primigravida presents with lower abdominal pain at 14 weeks' gestation. There is no history of vaginal bleeding or dysuria. She has had an episode of vomiting in the morning. On examination her temperature is 37.8°C. There is tenderness in her lower abdomen, particularly the right lower quadrant. Vaginal examination reveals a closed cervix with no bleeding. Blood results are: haemoglobin 11.7 gm/dl, white blood cell count 17.0 cells/mm³, CRP 100 units, AST 30 IU, GGT 17 IU, ALP 150 IU, bilirubin 22 mg/dl, amylase 50 IU and serum albumin 25 g/dl.

C   Appendicitis commonly presents in the early second trimester in young mothers. The classical signs might be absent in pregnancy.

13 Gastrointestinal disorders in pregnancy

Answers: H C F

A 30-year-old woman who has a longstanding history of Crohn's disease is admitted at 28 weeks' gestation in her first pregnancy with multiple fistulae around the anus, which are associated with abscess formation.

H   Surgical treatment for abscess associated with perianal Crohn's disease is generally limited to the drainage and control of sepsis.

A 32-year-old pregnant woman presents with a painful perianal lump of 4 days' duration in the third trimester. She is known to have had problems with haemorrhoids in the past. On examination there are tender prolapsed circumferential haemorrhoids.

C   Prolapsed circumferential haemorrhoids are generally treated with ice packs as surgical treatment is fraught with excessive bleeding.

A 34-year-old pregnant lady presents at 30 weeks' gestation with severe tenesmus and intermittent bleeding per rectum. Rigid sigmoidoscopy shows an inflamed rectum. Rectal biopsies have been reported to be suggestive of ulcerative colitis.

F   Colitis may be exacerbated in pregnancy. Initial treatment is with topical steroids/mesalazine in the form of enemas.

14 Thromboembolism/venous disorders

Answers: N D H

A 31-year-old woman presents at 34 weeks' gestation with a dull ache in her left calf. She is a smoker, and on examination there are superficial varicose veins present on both sides with localised left calf tenderness. Doppler studies show a loss of patency of the left long saphenous vein with a thrombus extending for 5 cm along the left popliteal fossa.

N   The treatment dose of enoxaparin needs to be commenced immediately.

A 31-year-old woman presents at 34 weeks' gestation with severe pain in both calves. The pain generally worsens over the day. On examination there are marked varicosities involving the long saphenous territory. Duplex examination shows bilateral saphenofemoral reflux. Doppler studies confirm normal patency of the deep venous system of both legs.

D   Surgical treatment is not indicated during pregnancy. Conservative management is recommended.

A 31-year-old woman presents at 34 weeks' gestation with a twin pregnancy with pain in her right calf. She is a smoker and her body mass index is 34 at booking.

On examination she has bilateral varicose veins and right-sided superficial thrombophlebitis. Doppler studies report normal patency of the deep venous system of both legs. She has a family history of antithrombin III deficiency.

H Prophylaxis can be given with low molecular weight heparin or heparin in high-risk situations after consulting the haematologist.

15 Syncope in pregnancy

Answers: F J A

A 30-year-old primigravid woman presents at 12 weeks' gestation. She is complaining of dizziness and vertigo. She states that she had a chest infection a week ago. On examination her dizziness is worse on turning her head. Her pulse and blood pressure are normal. She also has demonstrable nystagmus.

F Labyrinthitis is a complication of upper respiratory infection.

A 30-year-old lady who is in her second pregnancy attends the antenatal clinic for her booking. She complains of feeling dizzy after her booking blood tests. She has no prior history of dizziness. On examination her pulse rate is found to be 45 beats/minute, and her blood pressure is 120/76 mmHg. She has no neurological signs.

J Vasovagal symptoms are more common in pregnancy.

A 30-year-old lady presents in her second pregnancy at 34 weeks' gestation with dizziness. She is otherwise well with no other medical problems. She states that her dizziness is worse in the mornings and is relieved by rest. On examination her vital signs are normal. A full blood count demonstrates that her haemoglobin is 13.1 g/dL.

A Supine hypotension is often responsible for early-morning symptoms.

16 Thyroid diseases complicating pregnancy

Answers: D D I O

A 34-year-old primigravida is admitted to the antenatal ward. She is 18 weeks pregnant. She complains of a 2-day history of vomiting and a feeling that her heart has been beating faster on several occasions. On examination she looks anxious. She has a persistent pulse rate of 110 beats/minute and blood pressure of 140/70 mmHg. On examination of the hands she has a fine tremor. Thyroid function tests (TFTs) show a free thyroxine (T4) of 200 nmol/L (normal range 70–140 nmol/L), a tri-iodothyronine (T3) of 6 nmol/L (1.2–3.0 nmol/L) and a thyroid-stimulating hormone (TSH) level of 0.1 μ/L (0.5–5.0 nmol/L). The electrocardiograph shows sinus tachycardia.

D Graves' disease, if diagnosed during pregnancy, can be treated with propylthiouracil. However, initial acute-stage management would need beta-blockers and supportive measures.

A 27-year-old lady presents 12 weeks after the birth of her first child. She is complaining of a painful swelling in her neck and her heart beating faster. On examination her pulse is 110 beats/minute. Her thyroid gland is enlarged and non-tender. Her TFTs show a free T4 of 180 nmol/L (70–140 nmol/L), a T3 of 8 nmol/L (1.2–3.0 nmol/L) and a TSH of 0.28 μ/L (0.5–5.0 nmol/L). Radioactive iodine uptake shows a low uptake into the thyroid gland.

D   Postpartum thyroiditis usually recovers spontaneously. If, however, the hyperthyroid state merits treatment, this should be aimed at symptom relief, which would be beta-blockers and not antithyroid drugs.

A 27-year-old woman presents at 24 weeks' gestation in her first pregnancy. She complains of a swelling in her neck. On examination the thyroid gland is enlarged and tender. She states that she had a sore throat and generalized malaise 2 weeks ago. Her TFTs show a free T4 of 160 nmol/L (70–140 nmol/L), a T3 of 6 nmol/L (1.2–3.0 nmol/L) and a TSH of 0.1 μ/L (0.5–5.0 nmol/L).

I   De Quervain's thyroiditis is usually self-limiting.

A 27-year-old woman is referred to antenatal clinic at 28 weeks' gestation in her first pregnancy. The community midwife has measured the symphysis–fundus height at 24 cm. The woman is known to be hypothyroid secondarily to Graves' disease and is currently taking thyroxine supplementation. On examination the symphysis–fundus height measures 25 cm. The woman's TFTs show a free T4 of 86 nmol/L (70–140 nmol/L), a T3 of 2.1 (1.2–3.0 nmol/L) and a TSH of 2.2 μ/L (0.5–5.0 nmol/L) level. Ultrasound demonstrates a fetal goitre with fetal heart rate of 200 beats/minute. AC (abdominal circumference) and HC (head circumference) are on the third centile. Umbilical artery Doppler studies are normal.

O   Antithyroid drugs need to be given to the mother along with thyroxine to prevent fetal/neonatal thyrotoxicosis.

17 Chest pain in pregnancy

Answers: G K N E

A 46-year-old lady who conceived with ovum donation presents at 34 weeks' gestation with a sudden onset of central chest pain and breathlessness. She smokes about 15 cigarettes a day. On examination, her pulse is 98 beats/minute and her blood pressure (BP) is 100/70 mmHg. The symphysis–fundus height is appropriate for gestation, and the fetal heart is heard normally. The chest X-ray is reported to be normal. An electrocardiogram (ECG) shows a sinus rhythm with T wave inversion noted in leads III, aVL and aVF.

G   The history of ovum donation would suggest a history of premature ovarian failure. This, in combination with smoking, increases the risk of coronary heart disease. The ECG changes are suggestive of an inferior wall ischaemia.

A 26-year-old woman presents at 27 weeks' gestation in her second pregnancy with severe chest pain that radiates to her back. Her height is 170 cm and she has been noted to have hypermobile joints. On examination she looks unwell with a pulse rate of 136 beats/minute and a BP of 76/46 mmHg. The chest X-ray is reported to be normal. An ECG shows sinus rhythm with a rate of 128 beats/minute.

K   A high index of suspicion for this life-threatening condition is needed in people with marfanoid features.

A 32-year-old Asian lady who has recently moved to the UK presents at 20 weeks' gestation in her third pregnancy with left-sided chest pain. She describes becoming increasingly breathless over the past 4 weeks. She gives a recent history of easy fatigability and lassitude. On examination her pulse rate is 88 beats/minute and her BP is 96/70 mmHg. Auscultation of the heart reveals muffled heart sounds. An ECG shows low-voltage complexes.

N   Pericardial effusion due to tuberculosis can present in this manner. The signs are suggestive of pericardial effusion.

A 30-year-old schoolteacher presents at 30 weeks' gestation with right-sided chest pain, which is made worse on coughing. She also complains of a productive cough. On examination her pulse is 110 beats/minute and her BP is 100/76 mmHg. Her temperature is 38°C. The heart sounds are normal, and breath sounds are diminished on the right side. The chest X-ray shows a ground-glass appearance on the right side.

E   A combination of fever, productive cough and chest pain with X-ray changes is suggestive of pneumonia.

18 Diabetes in pregnancy

Answers: H G A D

A 27-year-old lady is 26 weeks pregnant in her second pregnancy. In her first pregnancy she had an emergency caesarean section for failure to progress. The baby weighed 4.0 kg. She has an oral glucose tolerance test and her results are as follows: fasting glucose 7.2 mmol/L, 2-hour postprandial glucose 10.8 mmol/L.

H   The GTT is the standard way of assessing gestational diabetes.

A known insulin-dependent diabetic patient attends the combined clinic for follow-up and is found to have inadequately controlled glycaemia with an increasing glucose level.

G   The insulin requirement is likely to increase during pregnancy.

A woman with diet-controlled gestational diabetes mellitus is seen in the antenatal clinic at 33 weeks' gestation and found to have a symphysis–fundus height of 37 cm. Her blood sugar values over the last 2 weeks have been progressively increasing in spite of good dietary restrictions.

A   Insulin administration should be commenced.

A 30-year-old lady who had a stillbirth in her previous pregnancy has been found to have undiagnosed diabetes. She is currently on oral hypoglycaemic agents, with good glycaemic control, and attends for prepregnancy counselling. What is the appropriate next step?

D   The glycated haemoglobin level is a good indicator of glycaemic status.

19 Palpitations in pregnancy

Answers: B K G A

A 35-year-old lady who is para 2 presents with palpitations. She has associated non-proteinuric hypertension inadequately controlled by methyldopa. She is complaining of intermittent headaches and sweating.

B   The intermittent nature of the symptoms is suggestive of phaeochromocytoma; 24-hour urinary catecholamines will confirm the diagnosis.

A 27-year-old anxious-looking primigravid woman presents at 18 weeks' gestation with palpitations and tremors. Her haemoglobin level is 112 mg/dl. An electrocardiogram shows sinus tachycardia.

K   The history is suggestive of thyrotoxicosis. Thyroid function tests are necessary for diagnosis.

A 32-year-old lady of oriental origin presents at 18 weeks' gestation with palpitations. She has a long history of breathlessness. She also recollects having swollen joints and fever in childhood.

G   Rheumatic heart disease is still common in developing countries. Penicillin prophylaxis is needed. Mitral stenosis is the common manifestation of longstanding disease leading to atrial fibrillation. This can be aggravated in pregnancy.

A healthy pregnant woman attends for her booking at 34 weeks' gestation. She mentions occasional palpitations with no other associated symptoms. Her haemoglobin is 12.1 g/dL.

A   Palpitations can be physiological in pregnancy due to an increased cardiovascular demand and workload.

20 Vomiting/liver function tests in pregnancy

Answers: G B C D F M

A 23-year-old primigravida presents at 36 weeks' gestation with severe generalised itching and sleeplessness. Liver function tests (LFTs) are as follows: bilirubin 10 mg/dl, aspartate aminotransferase (AST) 35 IU, alanine aminotransferase (ALT) 40 IU and alkaline phosphatase 1000 IU. What is the most likely diagnosis?

G   Alkaline phosphatase can be elevated in normal pregnancy.

A 28-year-old lady who is para 2 presents at 12 weeks' gestation with fever, malaise and vomiting. LFTs arranged by her GP are as follows: bilirubin 24 mg/dl, AST 100 IU, ALT 120 IU and alkaline phosphatase 800 IU. What is the most likely diagnosis?

B   Fever and malaise along with jaundice are generally indicative of viral hepatitis.

A 32-year-old primipara presents at 32 weeks' gestation with severe itching involving her palms and soles. LFTs are as follows: bilirubin 10 mg/dl, AST 50 IU, ALT 58 IU, alkaline phosphatase 660 IU and bile acids 26 mg/dl. What is the most likely diagnosis?

C   Severe itching in the third trimester involving the palms and soles is character-istic of obstetric cholestasis.

A 19-year-old girl presents at 32 weeks' gestation with nausea, vomiting, abdominal pain and severe malaise of 2 days' duration. On examination her Glasgow coma score is 11. She was diagnosed with mild pre-eclampsia at 28 weeks' gestation. LFTs show bilirubin 24 mg/dl, AST 100 IU and ALT 120 IU. What is the most likely diagnosis?

D   Acute fatty liver of pregnancy can present as hepatic encephalopathy. HELLP syndrome is a differential diagnosis, which is excluded by normal platelets.

A 25-year-old woman presents at 18 weeks' gestation with severe bloodstained vomiting and tiredness. On examination she is dehydrated. LFTs are as follows: bilirubin 10 mg/dl, AST 50 IU, ALT 45 IU, alkaline phosphatase 480 IU. Her haematocrit is 0.48 l/L, and urine analysis shows ketones. What is the most likely diagnosis?

F   Ketonuria and haematemesis are suggestive of hyperemesis gravidarum.

A 24-year-old pregnant lady presents at 20 weeks' gestation with severe abdominal pain and dehydration. She has recently been diagnosed with gallstones. LFTs are as follows: bilirubin 25 mg/dl, amylase 1000 IU, AST 60 IU, ALT 68 IU and alkaline phosphatase 1500 IU. What is the most likely diagnosis?

M   Gallstone-induced pancreatitis can present rarely in pregnancy.

21 Medications in pregnancy

Answers: C N K

A 32-week primigravid lady is admitted to the labour ward with irregular tightenings. She denies any history of bleeding per vaginum or draining. She is an ex-smoker who recently quit smoking. There are no significant medical or surgical problems. On examination the presentation is cephalic and the cervix is posterior and closed. Urine analysis is negative. The woman is then given the stat dose of a tocolytic, after which she develops a severe headache, hypotension and flushing.

C   Nifedipine is associated with side-effects.

A 38-year-old primigravida is currently 22 weeks pregnant and is being seen in the antenatal clinic following her anomaly scan. She is known to have epilepsy, for which she is on medication. The initial scan was incomplete as the facial anatomy was difficult to achieve. A subsequent detailed scan confirms a cleft lip. The woman's last episode of fits was a year ago.

N   Phenytoin is associated with oral clefting.

A 22-year-old lady is admitted to the labour ward at 34 weeks' gestation. She was diagnosed with pre-eclampsia and was started on medication 2 weeks ago. She is feeling low and depressed but denies any history of headache or visual disturbances. On examination her reflexes are normal and there is an adequately grown fetus. Her blood pressure is 130/76 mmHg and there is 1+ proteinuria. Her renal function and liver function tests are normal.

K   One of the main side-effects of methyldopa is low mood.

22 Psychiatric disorders in pregnancy and the puerperium

Answers: M E G

A 23-year-old woman who has had a normal delivery 12 hours earlier is noted by the ward staff to be having difficulties sleeping, is overactive and expresses feelings of excitement.

M   Many symptoms in the postnatal period may mimic psychiatric disorders, and a detailed history and careful evaluation are necessary.

A 23-year-old woman presents at the booking clinic. She is 7 weeks pregnant in her first pregnancy and has been referred by the community midwife for consultant care. She feels well in herself and says that a specific voice has been speaking to her every morning instructing her to do things. She is not on any medication.

E   Auditory hallucinations, thought withdrawal, insertion and interruption thought broadcasting, delusional perception and feelings or actions experienced as made or influenced by external agents are considered as first-rank symptoms of schizophrenia.

A 40-year-old woman presents on the fifth day after a normal delivery. Her husband brought her in to Accident and Emergency after he noticed an abrupt change in her behaviour. He describes her as confused, restless and expressing thoughts of self-harm.

G   The prevalence of postnatal depression is about 10 per cent, but severe depression with suicidal thoughts is relatively less common. Immediate psychiatric evaluation, preferably in a mother and baby unit, is necessary.

23 Headache

Answers: F K P J

A 32-year-old lady is admitted via the Accident and Emergency unit with sudden severe unilateral right-sided headache at 12 weeks' gestation. She is noted to have swelling around her right eye. Her blood pressure is normal and there are no focal neurological signs. There is no history of migraines.

F   Cluster headache is more common in men than women, but periorbital oedema and unilateral presentation are typical.

A 38-year-old lady presents to the labour ward with headache. She works as a manager and is currently 24 weeks pregnant. She describes it as a squeezing type of pain in her forehead. Her blood pressure and neurological examination are normal.

K   Tension headache is typically described as a tight band or squeezing type of headache and is related to stress. Simple analgesics help in relieving the pain.

A 39-year-old lady attends the day unit with headache. She is 26 weeks pregnant and was on captopril, which was later converted to methyldopa at booking. Nifedipine has recently been added to her medication. There is no proteinuria

and she denies any history of visual disturbances. On examination her reflexes are normal.

P   Severe headaches with flushing are common with nifedipine.

A 23-year-old primigravida is seen in the day unit for severe headache of insidious origin and associated vomiting without any nausea. She is 28 weeks pregnant in her second pregnancy and has no proteinuria. Her blood pressure is 90/60 mmHg and her pulse rate 78 beats/minute. There is no significant medical or surgical history. Initial blood investigations are normal. Fundoscopy reveals bilateral papilloedema.

J   Intracranial symptoms are more difficult to differentiate in pregnancy.

Section 4: Labour and puerperium

24 Mechanism of labour

25 Third-stage complications

26 Intrapartum care

27 Maternal collapse

28 Shoulder dystocia

29 Postpartum haemorrhage

30 Intrauterine death

31 Preterm labour

32 Perinatal injuries

33 Malpresentations

34 Labour risks

35 Tests on the labour suite

QUESTIONS

24 Mechanism of labour

A descent
B extension
C engagement
D flexion
E external rotation
F restitution
G internal rotation
H none of the above

For each description below, choose the **single** most appropriate answer from the above list of options. Each option may be used once, more than once, or not at all.

1   After the head delivers through the vulva, it immediately aligns with the fetal shoulders.

2   The occiput escapes from underneath the symphysis pubis, which acts as a fulcrum.

3   The anterior shoulder lies inferior to the symphysis pubis and delivers first, and the posterior shoulder delivers subsequently.

4   When the widest part of the presenting part has passed successfully through the pelvic inlet.

Answers: see page 63.

25 Third-stage complications

A   postpartum cardiomyopathy
B   thromboembolism
C   amniotic fluid embolism
D   vaginal tear
E   uterine inversion
F   atonic postpartum haemorrhage
G   eclampsia
H   epilepsy
I   cervical trauma
J   fat embolism
K   anaphylaxis
L   postpartum collapse
M   torsion of an ovarian cyst
N   thrombosis of the sagittal sinus
O   subarachnoid haemorrhage

For each description below, choose the **single** most appropriate answer from the above list of options. Each option may be used once, more than once, or not at all.

1   A 32-year-old woman in her first pregnancy has had a low-cavity forceps delivery for prolonged second stage under spinal anaesthesia. After delivery she is noted to have excessive vaginal bleeding. On examination she is noted to have excessive blood loss and to appear pale. The pulse is noted to be 110 beats/minute and blood pressure 120/70 mmHg. Abdominal examination reveals that the uterus is well contracted. Examination of the placenta confirms it to be complete.

2   A 32-year-old in her third pregnancy is admitted to the hospital with severe abdominal pain. She was evaluated for a suspicious adnexal mass during the antenatal period. She collapsed in the bathroom on the first postnatal day.

3   A 28-year-old para 5 had a quick labour. The baby weighed 4.3 kg. Examination of the placenta was noted to be complete. On examination she was observed to be pale and clammy. The maternal pulse was noted to demonstrate a tachycardia of 110 beats/minute and her blood pressure was 100/60 mmHg. The perineum was noted to be intact, but heavy vaginal bleeding was observed.

4   A 36-year-old woman in her second pregnancy had an uneventful first and second stage of labour. The placenta was delivered by continuous cord traction. Shortly after delivery of the placenta she complained of severe abdominal pain and collapsed. On examination her pulse was noted to be 40 beats/minute and her blood pressure was 50/30 mmHg. On abdominal examination the uterus was not palpable.

Answers: see page 63.

26 Intrapartum care

A category II caesarean section
B artificial rupture of the membranes
C continuous cardiotocography (CTG)
D elective caesarean section
E fetal blood sampling
F fetal scalp electrode
G ventouse delivery
H repeat fetal blood sampling in 30 minutes
I category III caesarean section
J await normal delivery
K oxytocin for augmentation
L category I caesarean section
M internal podalic version
N repeat fetal blood sampling in 15 minutes

For each description below, choose the **single** most appropriate answer from the above list of options. Each option may be used once, more than once, or not at all.

1 A 25-year-old primigravida has fetal bradycardia in the second stage of labour. She has no pain relief and has been pushing for the past 30 minutes. The fetal head is in the left occipitoposterior position with head below the ischial spines.

2 A 27-year-old woman in her first pregnancy who is a heavy smoker is being induced at 38 weeks' gestation for intrauterine growth restriction and oligo-hydramnios. On vaginal examination the cervix is 5 cm dilated. Review of the CTG shows a baseline of 140 beats/minute, reduced variability and decelerations. The decelerations last for longer than 15 seconds, and the nadir occurs after the contraction.

3 A 32-year-old woman in her first pregnancy presents in spontaneous labour at 40 weeks and 4 days with rupture of membranes. On vaginal examination the cervix is found to be 7 cm dilated. Meconium-stained liquor is noted. Review of the admission CTG after 20 minutes is uninterpretable due to areas of loss of contact.

4 A 28-year-old woman in her second pregnancy has been admitted for induction of labour for postmaturity, and oxytocin augmentation has been commenced. Assessment of the partogram has revealed satisfactory progress. Medical review of the CTG prompted a fetal blood sample 30 minutes ago, which demonstrated a pH of 7.25. On vaginal examination the cervical dilatation was noted to be 9 cm, and the CTG remained similar.

5 A 32-year-old woman who has had an uncomplicated antenatal period is admitted in spontaneous labour at term with good progress. She is on continuous monitoring due to audible fetal heart decelerations heard on intermittent auscultation in the second stage of labour. The CTG shows a baseline of 140 beats/minute,

a variability of 7–10, no accelerations and decelerations with spontaneous recovery, and shouldering. She has been pushing for the last 10 minutes with the fetal head in the +1 station in the right occipitoposterior position.

Answers: see page 64.

27 Maternal collapse

A pulmonary embolism
B amniotic fluid embolism
C eclamptic fit
D massive placental abruption
E epilepsy
F postpartum haemorrhage
G disseminated intravascular coagulation
H subarachnoid haemorrhage
I aortic stenosis
J hyperventilation
K migraine
L vasovagal attack
M hypoglycaemia
N aortic dissection
O cerebral haemorrhage

For each description below, choose the **single** most appropriate answer from the above list of options. Each option may be used once, more than once, or not at all.

1 A 39-year-old woman in her first pregnancy is being induced for symphysis pubis dysfunction at 38 weeks. During the first stage of labour she was noted to have uterine hyperstimulation, which was corrected by reducing the oxytocin infusion. She was delivered later by lower-segment caesarean section for a sub-optimal cardiotocogram (CTG). Two hours post delivery she complained of shortness of breath. On examination she was noted to be cyanotic and her pulse was 100 beats/minute. A chest X-ray was performed that demonstrated a bilateral ground-glass appearance with an impaired coagulation profile.

2 A 22-year-old in her first pregnancy presents to Accident and Emergency at 14 weeks of gestation with severe sudden occipital headache. She had projectile vomiting prior to arrival. After admission her score on the Glasgow Coma Scale falls to 3.

3 A 26-year-old lady who had a spontaneous delivery 3 days ago is found collapsed at home. In her history she had been noted to have had pre-eclampsia in this pregnancy.

4 A 32-year-old woman in her second pregnancy collapses in the day assessment unit at 34 weeks' gestation. She is a known insulin-dependent diabetic. Her insulin dose was increased a week ago because of persistently high blood sugar readings. She complained of sweating and palpitations soon after arrival in the clinic.

Answers: see page 65.

28 Shoulder dystocia

A   McRoberts manoeuvre
B   suprapubic pressure
C   episiotomy
D   McRoberts manoeuvre and suprapubic pressure
E   category I caesarean section
F   Zavanelli's technique
G   release of the posterior arm
H   pelvic manoeuvres
I   symphysiotomy
J   cleidotomy
K   call for assistance
L   move onto all fours
M   do nothing
N   elective caesarean section
O   destructive procedures

For each description below, choose the **single** most appropriate answer from the above list of options. Each option may be used once, more than once, or not at all.

1   A 25-year-old nurse from the Philippines developed gestational diabetes in her first pregnancy, which is well controlled. She was induced at term and has had a prolonged first and second stage of labour. The baby's head is delivered spontaneously with prior episiotomy, and the turtling sign is observed. Help has been summoned. What is the appropriate next step?

2   A 26-year-old woman in her second pregnancy has progressed normally in the first and second stages of labour. A forceps delivery is undertaken due to a sub-optimal CTG. There is difficulty in delivering the fetal shoulder. Help has been summoned. Suprapubic pressure and the McRoberts procedure have been unsuccessful. What is the appropriate next step?

3   A 31-year-old in her second pregnancy has had an uneventful antenatal period under midwifery care and opted for a home delivery. She has laboured at home and has a shoulder dystocia after delivery of the head. An ambulance has been summoned. The McRoberts, suprapubic pressure and pelvic manoeuvres have been unsuccessful. What is the appropriate next step?

4   A 32-year-old Chinese lady with short stature develops gestational diabetes. She is being induced at 38 weeks for fetal macrosomia. After delivery of the head shoulder dystocia is diagnosed with both fetal shoulders above the pelvic brim. What is the appropriate next step?

Answers: see page 65.

29 Postpartum haemorrhage

A summon help
B methotrexate
C bimanual compression
D fresh frozen plasma
E B Lynch suturing
F laparotomy/hysterectomy
G 40 units of oxytocin in 500 ml of normal saline
H intramuscular carboprost
I repeat Syntometrine
J examination under anaesthesia
K examination of the placenta
L intravenous access
M internal iliac artery ligation
N broad-spectrum antibiotics
O uterine packing

For each description below, choose the **single** most appropriate answer from the above list of options. Each option may be used once, more than once, or not at all.

1 A 27-year-old multiparous woman has a rapid delivery soon after arriving in the delivery suite. After delivery of the placenta she is noted to have heavy vaginal bleeding. Help has been summoned. What is the most appropriate next step?

2 A 22-year-old woman in her first pregnancy is noted to have prolonged first and second stages of labour. She was induced at 38 weeks' gestation for pre-eclampsia and was augmented with oxytocin. She bleeds heavily after the third stage and already has two intravenous lines inserted. Help has been summoned and an oxytocin infusion has been set up. Abdominal examination demonstrates a relaxed uterus. What is the most appropriate next step?

3 A 38-year-old lady has had a forceps delivery for prolonged second stage. The placenta is noted to be complete on examination. She has a massive postpartum haemorrhage (PPH). Help has been summoned and intravenous access obtained. Syntometrine has been given. On examination the uterus is well contracted. What is the most appropriate next step?

4 A 25-year-old woman in her first pregnancy is being induced for unexplained intrauterine death at 37 weeks' gestation. She has received three doses of vaginal prostaglandin and been augmented with oxytocin infusion. She has a PPH. Intravenous access has already been secured. On examination the uterus is well contracted and the placenta is noted to be complete. Blood investigations reveal a haemoglobin level of 11.2 g/dL, and the activated partial thromboplastin time is 70 seconds with a control of 32 seconds. What is the most appropriate management option?

Answers: see page 66.

30 Intrauterine death

A   immediate caesarean section
B   oxytocin augmentation
C   coagulation screening
D   intravenous access and fresh frozen plasma
E   prostaglandin F2 alpha
F   artificial rupture of membranes
G   ultrasound
H   oral misoprostol followed by vaginal prostaglandins
I   counselling
J   control hypertension
K   mifepristone followed by misoprostol
L   vaginal prostaglandin E2
M   single-dose misoprostol
N   admission, intravenous access and coagulation screen
O   extra-amniotic saline infusion

For each description below, choose the **single** most appropriate answer from the above list of options. Each option may be used once, more than once, or not at all.

1   A 27-year-old primigravida attends the delivery suite with a history of diminished fetal movements for 2 days. She is a smoker with no other risk factors. On examination the uterus is not tense or tender, and the fetal heart is not heard on auscultation. Intrauterine fetal death is confirmed later by ultrasound. She is extremely distressed and demands a caesarean section. Her observations are normal.

2   A 26-year old para 0 + 3 presents at 28 weeks' gestation feeling unwell. She has had two previous first-trimester miscarriages, and her last pregnancy ended in a miscarriage at 18 weeks. She is on oral aspirin. On examination her blood pressure (BP) is 140/100 mmHg and there is 3+ proteinuria on urinalysis. Her booking BP is noted to be 120/80 mmHg. An ultrasound scan confirms fetal death. She wants to initiate the delivery process immediately.

3   A 32-year-old woman in her fourth pregnancy attends the delivery suite at 36 weeks' gestation with abdominal pain and bleeding. On physical examination the uterus is tense and tender to palpation. Her BP is 100/60 mmHg and her pulse rate 90 beats/minute. The fetal heart is absent and this is confirmed by ultrasound. On vaginal examination the cervix is 4 cm dilated and the woman is contracting 3 in 10.

4   A 30-year-old woman in her second pregnancy presents at 32 weeks' gestation with heavy vaginal blood loss (estimated blood loss 1000 mL). She has had a previous caesarean section for breech presentation. An ultrasound scan performed at 31 weeks' gestation demonstrated that the placenta was covering part of the internal os. On examination her BP is 90/60 mmHg and her pulse is 98 beats/minute. There is no audible fetal heart, which is confirmed by ultrasound.

Answers: see page 67.

31 Preterm labour

A in utero transfer
B dexamethasone
C erythromycin
D a loading dose of intravenous benzylpenicillin and 4-hourly doses during labour
E caesarean section
F cervical cerclage
G counselling about neonatal outcome
H intravenous antibiotics
I cervical ultrasound
J oral metronidazole
K a tocolytic
L vaginal swabs
M home uterine activity monitoring
N midstream urine cultures
O thyrotrophin-releasing hormone

For each description below, choose the **single** most appropriate answer from the above list of options. Each option may be used once, more than once, or not at all.

1 A 22-year-old para 2 presents to the delivery suite at 32 weeks' gestation with abdominal pain and dysuria. Her urine dipstick shows white blood cells and nitrites. Midstream urine results are awaited. On speculum examination the cervix is found to be 3 cm dilated with intact membranes.

2 A 24-year-old woman in her first pregnancy attends the day assessment unit at 31 weeks' gestation with a watery vaginal discharge of 2 days' duration. On speculum examination there is clear liquor draining. She is not in labour and has received steroids a week previously for threatened preterm labour.

3 A 34-year-old primipara attends the delivery suite with periodic abdominal pain at 33 weeks' gestation. She has diabetes, which is poorly controlled on insulin. On examination the cervix is 2 cm dilated. She has been given the first dose of steroids.

4 A 31-year-old para 2 lady attends the day assessment unit with a history of increased vaginal discharge at 32 weeks' gestation. She is not in labour, and there is no evidence of preterm rupture of the membranes. A high vaginal swab shows bacterial vaginosis.

Answers: see page 68.

32 Perineal injuries

A repair by an overlap technique with non-absorbable suture material with intermittent sutures to the vaginal mucosa, perineal muscle and subcutaneous layer
B offer elective caesarean section
C defunctioning colostomy and elective rectal mucosal repair 6 weeks later
D complete the repair under local anaesthesia
E repair by an overlap technique with absorbable sutures and intermittent sutures to the vaginal mucosa, perineal muscle and subcutaneous layer
F broad-spectrum antibiotics
G pelvic floor exercises
H repair the rectal mucosal defect before sphincter repair
I repair the anal sphincter followed by the rectal mucosa
J endoanal ultrasound
K a defunctioning colostomy and simultaneous rectal mucosal repair
L appropriate repair in theatre under regional anaesthesia
M repair by an overlap technique with polydixanone sutures with continuous sutures to vaginal mucosa, perineal muscle and subcutaneous layer
N stool softeners
O barium enema

For each description below, choose the **single** most appropriate answer from the above list of options. Each option may be used once, more than once, or not at all.

1 A 29-year-old lady undergoes trial instrumental delivery in theatre for a sub-optimal cardiotocograph. She sustains a third-degree perineal tear.

2 A 22-year-old lady has a prolonged second stage of labour, and the baby delivers face to pubis. On examination there is complete disruption of the anal sphincter and a 2 cm defect in the rectal mucosa.

3 A 36-year-old lady has undergone a forceps delivery after a prolonged second stage. On examination there was a second-degree perineal tear that was repaired at this time. A week later she presents with a smelly vaginal discharge. On vaginal examination there is a 1 cm buttonhole defect involving rectal mucosa in the upper vagina. You are being called to review a tear being repaired by the midwife due to difficulties. On examination a third-degree tear is found.

Answers: see page 68.

33 Malpresentations

A category I caesarean section
B breech extraction
C admit and observation
D category IV caesarean section
E stabilising induction
F expectant management
G internal podalic version
H category II caesarean section
I vaginal breech delivery
J oxytocin augmentation
K induction at 36 weeks
L artificial rupture of membranes
M Lovset's manoeuvre
N external cephalic version
O category III caesarean section
P destructive procedures

For each description below, choose the **single** most appropriate answer from the above list of options. Each option may be used once, more than once, or not at all.

1 A 30-year-old primigravida attends the delivery suite at 39 weeks' gestation in established labour. On vaginal examination she is 4 cm dilated with a foot presentation.

2 A community midwife refers a 34-year-old in her fifth pregnancy for an unstable lie at 37 weeks' gestation. On clinical examination the fetus is presenting transversely with an adequate liquor volume. There is no uterine activity, and vaginal examination reveals a closed cervix.

3 A 30-year-old woman in her first pregnancy presents at 36 weeks' gestation in spontaneous labour. On abdominal examination she is contracting 3 in 10. On vaginal examination the cervix is 3 cm dilated. The vertex is at −3 cm above the ischial spines with a fetal limb felt alongside the vertex.

4 A community midwife refers a 27-year-old woman in her first pregnancy at 37 weeks' gestation for a suspected breech presentation. She is fit and healthy. Breech presentation is confirmed by ultrasound scan.

Answers: see page 69.

34 Labour risks

A   1:120
B   1:200
C   1:50
D   90:100
E   1:270
F   1:1000
G   3:100
H   1:100
I   50:100
J   1:1500
K   22:100
L   7:1000

For each description below, choose the **single** most appropriate answer from the above list of options. Each option may be used once, more than once, or not at all.

1   A 32-year-old woman is admitted at 40 weeks' gestation from home in labour. It was noted on a 28-week scan that the fetus was in the breech presentation. What is the risk of the fetus remaining breech?

2   A 23-year-old woman is admitted in labour. She is in her second pregnancy, her first having been an elective caesarean section for breech presentation. What is the risk of scar rupture?

3   A 30-year-old lady presents at term in spontaneous labour in her third pregnancy. She had previously had two spontaneous vaginal deliveries. She has a prelabour rupture of membranes and a prolonged first stage in labour. The head is 3/5th palpable via the abdomen. Vaginal examination shows the presence of the bregma in the centre of the cervix, which is 4 cm dilated. What is the risk of this presentation in labour?

4   A 27-year-old primigravida presents with a history of spontaneous rupture of membranes at 36 weeks' gestation. She is known to have had an amniotic fluid index of 27 cm on a previous scan. Speculum examination shows the presence of a loop of cord in the vagina. What is the incidence of this complication?

Answers: see page 70.

35 Tests on the labour suite

A full blood count (FBC)
B FBC/group and save
C cardiotocogram (CTG)
D speculum examination
E Apt test
F expectant management
G ultrasound examination
H vaginal examination
I FBC/urea and electrolytes/liver function tests/clotting
J electrocardiogram (ECG)
K arterial blood gases
L clotting screen
M FBC/C-reactive protein
N urinalysis
O midstream urine analysis

For each description below, choose the **single** most appropriate answer from the above list of options. Each option may be used once, more than once, or not at all.

1 A 40-year-old woman is admitted to the labour suite at 38 weeks. She has required infertility treatment. An ultrasound scan at 30 weeks had demonstrated a succenturiate lobe on the scan. She complains of a small vaginal bleed after spontaneous rupture of the fetal membranes. The admission CTG shows reduced variability and unprovoked decelerations. What would the most appropriate initial investigation be?

2 A 24-year old primigravida is referred by the community midwife at 32 weeks' gestation with raised blood pressure. Her blood pressure measures 150/96 mmHg with 2+ of proteinuria. She feels well in herself but has been experiencing severe pain in the epigastric region for the past few days. What is the most appropriate initial investigation?

3 A 24-year-old primigravida presents to the delivery suite with abdominal pain of a few hours' duration. She denies any history of bleeding or leaking but has been experiencing urinary frequency for the past week. The admission CTG is reassuring, with evidence of regular uterine activity over 40 minutes.

4 A 39-year-old lady is being induced for post dates. Her blood pressure was found to be elevated in the last few weeks of pregnancy with no significant proteinuria. She is complaining of palpitations and breathlessness. Her pulse is 98 beats/minute, and her blood pressure is found to be 130/70 mmHg. What is the most appropriate initial investigation?

Answers: see page 70.

ANSWERS

24 Mechanism of labour

Answers: F B H C

After the head delivers through the vulva, it immediately aligns with the fetal shoulders.

F   Restitution is the passive movement of shoulders to align with the head after passage through the vulva.

The occiput escapes from underneath the symphysis pubis, which acts as a fulcrum.

B   Extension of fetal head to complete the process of delivery of the fetal head.

The anterior shoulder lies inferior to the symphysis pubis and delivers first, and the posterior shoulder delivers subsequently.

H   None. No terminology is assigned for this mechanism.

When the widest part of the presenting part has passed successfully through the pelvic inlet.

C   Engagement is when the widest part of the fetal head passes through the inlet.

The mechanism of labour refers to the series of changes that occur in the position and attitude of the fetus during its passage through the birth canal. The process involves engagement, descent, flexion, internal rotation, extension, restitution, external rotation and delivery of the shoulders and fetal body. Engagement is said to have occurred when the widest part of the presenting part has passed successfully through the pelvic inlet.

25 Third-stage complications

Answers: I M F E

A 32-year-old woman in her first pregnancy has had a low-cavity forceps delivery for prolonged second stage under spinal anaesthesia. After delivery she is noted to have excessive vaginal bleeding. On examination she is noted to have excessive blood loss and to appear pale. The pulse is noted to be 110 beats/minute and blood pressure 120/70 mmHg. Abdominal examination reveals that the uterus is well contracted. Examination of the placenta confirms it to be complete.

I   Cervical tears are a common cause of traumatic postpartum haemorrhage. Vaginal tears are common after rotational forceps delivery.

A 32-year-old in her third pregnancy is admitted to the hospital with severe abdominal pain. She was evaluated for a suspicious adnexal mass during the antenatal period. She collapsed in the bathroom on the first postnatal day.

M   Torsion of the ovarian cyst happens commonly after delivery due to laxity of the tissues.

A 28-year-old para 5 had a quick labour. The baby weighed 4.3 kg. Examination of the placenta was noted to be complete. On examination she was observed to be

pale and clammy. The maternal pulse was noted to demonstrate a tachycardia of 110 beats/minute and her blood pressure was 100/60 mmHg. The perineum was noted to be intact, but heavy vaginal bleeding was observed.

F   Atonic postpartum haemorrhage is the most likely cause of the shock.

A 36-year-old woman in her second pregnancy had an uneventful first and second stage of labour. The placenta was delivered by continuous cord traction. Shortly after delivery of the placenta she complained of severe abdominal pain and collapsed. On examination her pulse was noted to be 40 beats/minute and her blood pressure was 50/30 mmHg. On abdominal examination the uterus was not palpable.

E   Abdominal pain followed by collapse and a non-palpable uterus suggests uterine inversion.

26 Intrapartum care

Answers: G E F H J

A 25-year-old primigravida has fetal bradycardia in the second stage of labour. She has no pain relief and has been pushing for the past 30 minutes. The fetal head is in the left occipitoposterior position with head below the ischial spines.

G   This is the quickest method of delivery under the circumstances.

A 27-year-old woman in her first pregnancy who is a heavy smoker is being induced at 38 weeks' gestation for intrauterine growth restriction and oligohydramnios. On vaginal examination the cervix is 5 cm dilated. Review of the CTG shows a baseline of 140 beats/minute, reduced variability and decelerations. The decelerations last for longer than 15 seconds, and the nadir occurs after the contraction.

E   Persistent late deceleration is an indication for fetal blood sampling.

A 32-year-old woman in her first pregnancy presents in spontaneous labour at 40 weeks and 4 days with rupture of membranes. On vaginal examination the cervix is found to be 7 cm dilated. Meconium-stained liquor is noted. Review of the admission CTG after 20 minutes is uninterpretable due to areas of loss of contact.

F   If a poor trace is obtained by external monitoring, a fetal scalp electrode is needed. CTG should not be interpreted with loss of contact.

A 28-year-old woman in her second pregnancy has been admitted for induction of labour for postmaturity, and oxytocin augmentation has been commenced. Assessment of the partogram has revealed satisfactory progress. Medical review of the CTG prompted a fetal blood sample 30 minutes ago, which demonstrated a pH of 7.25. On vaginal examination the cervical dilatation was noted to be 9 cm, and the CTG remained similar.

H   Repeat fetal blood sampling is indicated in half an hour if the fetal blood pH is between 7.2 and 7.25.

A 32-year-old woman who has had an uncomplicated antenatal period is admitted in spontaneous labour at term with good progress. She is on continuous monitoring due to audible fetal heart decelerations heard on intermittent auscultation in the second stage of labour. The CTG shows a baseline of 140 beats/minute, a variability of 7–10, no accelerations and decelerations with spontaneous recovery, and shouldering. She has been pushing for the last 10 minutes with the fetal head in the +1 station in the right occipitoposterior position.

J   Variable decelerations are suggestive of cord compression, and early decelerations suggesting head compression are common in the second stage of labour. A normal baseline and variability are reassuring features. An absence of accelerations in labour is not pathological.

27 Maternal collapse

Answers: B H C M

A 39-year-old woman in her first pregnancy is being induced for symphysis pubis dysfunction at 38 weeks. During the first stage of labour she was noted to have uterine hyperstimulation, which was corrected by reducing the oxytocin infusion. She was delivered later by lower-segment caesarean section for a suboptimal cardiotocogram (CTG). Two hours post delivery she complained of shortness of breath. On examination she was noted to be cyanotic and her pulse was 100 beats/minute. A chest X-ray was performed that demonstrated a bilateral ground-glass appearance with an impaired coagulation profile.

B   Augmentation of labour is a risk factor, along with increasing age, hypertonic uterine contractions, uterine trauma and induction of labour.

A 22-year-old in her first pregnancy presents to Accident and Emergency at 14 weeks of gestation with severe sudden occipital headache. She had projectile vomiting prior to arrival. After admission her score on the Glasgow Coma Scale falls to 3.

H   The features are suggestive of subarachnoid haemorrhage and could be confirmed by a computed tomography scan.

A 26-year-old lady who had a spontaneous delivery 3 days ago is found collapsed at home. In her history she had been noted to have had pre-eclampsia in this pregnancy.

C   Forty per cent of eclamptic fits occur in the postnatal period. They can occur up to 10 days after delivery.

A 32-year-old woman in her second pregnancy collapses in the day assessment unit at 34 weeks' gestation. She is a known insulin-dependent diabetic. Her insulin dose was increased a week ago because of persistently high blood sugar readings. She complained of sweating and palpitations soon after arrival in the clinic.

M   Hypoglycaemia is a common reason for maternal collapse, especially in diabetes complicating pregnancy.

28 Shoulder dystocia

Answers: D H L F

A 25-year-old nurse from the Philippines developed gestational diabetes in her first pregnancy, which is well controlled. She was induced at term and has had a prolonged first and second stage of labour. The baby's head is delivered spont-aneously with prior episiotomy, and the turtling sign is observed. Help has been summoned. What is the appropriate next step?

D   The majority of babies are delivered by these manoeuvres.

A 26-year-old woman in her second pregnancy has progressed normally in the first and second stages of labour. A forceps delivery is undertaken due to a sub-optimal CTG. There is difficulty in delivering the fetal shoulder. Help has been summoned. Suprapubic pressure and the McRoberts procedure have been unsuccessful. What is the appropriate next step?

H   Pelvic manoeuvres such as delivery of the posterior shoulder and Wood's Cox screw manoeuvres are the next steps.

A 31-year-old in her second pregnancy has had an uneventful antenatal period under midwifery care and opted for a home delivery. She has laboured at home and has a shoulder dystocia after delivery of the head. An ambulance has been summoned. The McRoberts, suprapubic pressure and pelvic manoeuvres have been unsuccessful. What is the appropriate next step?

L   In the home set-up, repeating all the manoeuvres on all fours would be the most appropriate.

A 32-year-old Chinese lady with short stature develops gestational diabetes. She is being induced at 38 weeks for fetal macrosomia. After delivery of the head shoulder dystocia is diagnosed with both fetal shoulders above the pelvic brim. What is the appropriate next step?

F   Zavanelli's technique under general anaesthesia could be considered in true shoulder dystocia.

29 Postpartum haemorrhage

Answers: L C J D

A 27-year-old multiparous woman has a rapid delivery soon after arriving in the delivery suite. After delivery of the placenta she is noted to have heavy vaginal bleeding. Help has been summoned. What is the most appropriate next step?

L   Intravenous access in the form of two wide-bore cannulae is the first step in the management of postpartum haemorrhage.

A 22-year-old woman in her first pregnancy is noted to have prolonged first and second stages of labour. She was induced at 38 weeks' gestation for pre-eclampsia and was augmented with oxytocin. She bleeds heavily after the third stage and already has two intravenous lines inserted. Help has been summoned and an oxytocin infusion has been set up. Abdominal examination demonstrates a relaxed uterus. What is the most appropriate next step?

C   Bimanual compression would be the next step in managing atonic PPH. This decreases the blood loss by kinking the uterine arteries.

A 38-year-old lady has had a forceps delivery for prolonged second stage. The pla-centa is noted to be complete on examination. She has a massive postpartum haemorrhage (PPH). Help has been summoned and intravenous access obtained. Syntometrine has been given. On examination the uterus is well contracted. What is the most appropriate next step?

J   Examination under anaesthesia to rule out traumatic PPH is needed in this scenario. Traumatic postpartum haemorrhage should be kept in mind in all instrumental deliveries.

A 25-year-old woman in her first pregnancy is being induced for unexplained intrauterine death at 37 weeks' gestation. She has received three doses of vaginal prostaglandin and been augmented with oxytocin infusion. She has a PPH. Intravenous access has already been secured. On examination the uterus is well contracted and the placenta is noted to be complete. Blood investigations reveal a haemoglobin level of 11.2 g/dL, and the activated partial thromboplastin time is 70 seconds with a control of 32 seconds. What is the most appropriate management option?

D   Both intrauterine death and massive haemorrhage are known risk factors for disseminated intravascular coagulation.

30 Intrauterine death

Answers: I L N A

A 27-year-old primigravida attends the delivery suite with a history of diminished fetal movements for 2 days. She is a smoker with no other risk factors. On examination the uterus is not tense or tender, and the fetal heart is not heard on auscultation. Intrauterine fetal death is confirmed later by ultrasound. She is extremely distressed and demands a caesarean section. Her observations are normal.

I   Due to the extreme distress caused by the situation, the choice of discussing the options later should be offered to the mother if she is clinically stable.

A 26-year old para 0+3 presents at 28 weeks' gestation feeling unwell. She has had two previous first-trimester miscarriages, and her last pregnancy ended in a miscarriage at 18 weeks. She is on oral aspirin. On examination her blood pressure (BP) is 140/100 mmHg and there is 3+ proteinuria on urinalysis. Her booking BP is noted to be 120/80 mmHg. An ultrasound scan confirms fetal death. She wants to initiate the delivery process immediately.

L   Even though mifepristone and misoprostol have a shorter induction delivery time, vaginal prostaglandin E2 would be the best option in this situation.

A 32-year-old woman in her fourth pregnancy attends the delivery suite at 36 weeks' gestation with abdominal pain and bleeding. On physical examination the uterus is tense and tender to palpation. Her BP is 100/60 mmHg and her pulse rate 90 beats/minute. The fetal heart is absent and this is confirmed by ultrasound. On vaginal examination the cervix is 4 cm dilated and the woman is contracting 3 in 10.

N   If labour is established, watchful expectancy is appropriate.

A 30-year-old woman in her second pregnancy presents at 32 weeks' gestation with heavy vaginal blood loss (estimated blood loss 1000 mL). She has had a previous caesarean section for breech presentation. An ultrasound scan performed at 31 weeks' gestation demonstrated that the placenta was covering part of the internal os. On examination her BP is 90/60 mmHg and her pulse is 98 beats/minute. There is no audible fetal heart, which is confirmed by ultrasound.

A   Grade III placenta praevia is an absolute indication for caesarean section even in the presence of fetal death.

31 Preterm labour

Answers: B C K J

A 22-year-old para 2 presents to the delivery suite at 32 weeks' gestation with abdominal pain and dysuria. Her urine dipstick shows white blood cells and nitrites. Midstream urine results are awaited. On speculum examination the cervix is found to be 3 cm dilated with intact membranes.

B   Steroid administration improves perinatal outcome and is indicated up to 36 weeks' gestation.

A 24-year-old woman in her first pregnancy attends the day assessment unit at 31 weeks' gestation with a watery vaginal discharge of 2 days' duration. On speculum examination there is clear liquor draining. She is not in labour and has received steroids a week previously for threatened preterm labour.

C   Erythromycin has been shown to improve the perinatal outcome in preterm premature rupture of membranes (ORACLE).

A 34-year-old primipara attends the delivery suite with periodic abdominal pain at 33 weeks' gestation. She has diabetes, which is poorly controlled on insulin. On examination the cervix is 2 cm dilated. She has been given the first dose of steroids.

K   Atosiban, an oxytocin antagonist, could be considered in conditions in which beta-agonists are contraindicated.

A 31-year-old para 2 lady attends the day assessment unit with a history of increased vaginal discharge at 32 weeks' gestation. She is not in labour, and there is no evidence of preterm rupture of the membranes. A high vaginal swab shows bacterial vaginosis.

J   Oral metronidazole lowers the risk of preterm birth by 60 per cent in women with bacterial vaginosis.

32 Perineal injuries

Answers: M H K

A 29-year-old lady undergoes trial instrumental delivery in theatre for a suboptimal cardiotocograph. She sustains a third-degree perineal tear.

M   The anal sphincter complex can be repaired by either an end-to-end technique or an overlapping technique. A loose, continuous, non-locking suture technique is associated with less postoperative perineal pain compared with an interrupted technique.

A 22-year-old lady has a prolonged second stage of labour, and the baby delivers face to pubis. On examination there is complete disruption of the anal sphincter and a 2 cm defect in the rectal mucosa.

H Rectal mucosa should be repaired prior to the sphincter repair.

A 36-year-old lady has undergone a forceps delivery after a prolonged second stage. On examination there was a second-degree perineal tear that was repaired at this time. A week later she presents with a smelly vaginal discharge. On vaginal examination there is a 1 cm buttonhole defect involving rectal mucosa in the upper vagina. You are being called to review a tear being repaired by the midwife due to difficulties. On examination a third-degree tear is found.

K A defunctioning colostomy is needed for better healing and could be reversed in 6–12 weeks' time.

33 Malpresentations

Answers: H C F N

A 30-year-old primigravida attends the delivery suite at 39 weeks' gestation in established labour. On vaginal examination she is 4 cm dilated with a foot presentation.

H A footling breech presentation is best managed by caesarean section. However, as there is no immediate threat to the life of the mother or the fetus, this is a category II caesarean section.

A community midwife refers a 34-year-old in her fifth pregnancy for an unstable lie at 37 weeks' gestation. On clinical examination the fetus is presenting transversely with an adequate liquor volume. There is no uterine activity, and vaginal examination reveals a closed cervix.

C Eighty-five per cent of unstable lies will resolve spontaneously. Inpatient care is indicated to initiate immediate delivery in the event of spontaneous rupture of membranes and subsequent cord prolapse.

A 30-year-old woman in her first pregnancy presents at 36 weeks' gestation in spontaneous labour. On abdominal examination she is contracting 3 in 10. On vaginal examination the cervix is 3 cm dilated. The vertex is at –3 cm above the ischial spines with a fetal limb felt alongside the vertex.

F A compound presentation involving the limb alongside the vertex often resolves spontaneously with good uterine contractions. Watchful expectancy is needed.

A community midwife refers a 27-year-old woman in her first pregnancy at 37 weeks' gestation for a suspected breech presentation. She is fit and healthy. Breech presentation is confirmed by ultrasound scan.

N External cephalic version at term has a success rate of 65 per cent and should be offered to all women with an uncomplicated breech presentation after 37 weeks of gestation.

34 Labour risks

Answers: K L J B

A 32-year-old woman is admitted at 40 weeks' gestation from home in labour. It was noted on a 28-week scan that the fetus was in the breech presentation. What is the risk of the fetus remaining breech?

K   22% risk of persistent breech presentation has been found.

A 23-year-old woman is admitted in labour. She is in her second pregnancy, her first having been an elective caesarean section for breech presentation. What is the risk of scar rupture?

L   The risk of scar rupture in women undergoing a trial of labour after a previous elective caesarean section is 0.7 per cent.

A 30-year-old lady presents at term in spontaneous labour in her third pregnancy. She had previously had two spontaneous vaginal deliveries. She has a prelabour rupture of membranes and a prolonged first stage in labour. The head is 3/5th palpable via the abdomen. Vaginal examination shows the presence of the bregma in the centre of the cervix, which is 4 cm dilated. What is the risk of this presentation in labour?

J   The incidence of both brow and face presentation in labour is 1:1500.

A 27-year-old primigravida presents with a history of spontaneous rupture of membranes at 36 weeks' gestation. She is known to have had an amniotic fluid index of 27 cm on a previous scan. Speculum examination shows the presence of a loop of cord in the vagina. What is the incidence of this complication?

B   The risk of cord prolapse is 1:200.

35 Tests on the labour suite

Answers: B I D L

A 40-year-old woman is admitted to the labour suite at 38 weeks. She has required infertility treatment. An ultrasound scan at 30 weeks had demonstrated a succenturiate lobe on the scan. She complains of a small vaginal bleed after spontaneous rupture of the fetal membranes. The admission CTG shows reduced variability and unprovoked decelerations. What would the most appropriate initial investigation be?

B   Vaginal bleeding and a suboptimal CTG point towards vasa praevia.

A 24-year old primigravida is referred by the community midwife at 32 weeks' gestation with raised blood pressure. Her blood pressure measures 150/96 mmHg with 2+ of proteinuria. She feels well in herself but has been experiencing severe pain in the epigastric region for the past few days. What is the most appropriate initial investigation?

I   HELLP (haemolytic anaemia, elevated liver enzymes and low platelet count) syndrome needs to be suspected in women with pre-eclampsia complaining of epigastric pain.

A 24-year-old primigravida presents to the delivery suite with abdominal pain of a few hours' duration. She denies any history of bleeding or leaking but has been experiencing urinary frequency for the past week. The admission CTG is reassuring, with evidence of regular uterine activity over 40 minutes.

D   The appropriate investigation is speculum examination for cervical dilatation to establish the diagnosis of preterm labour.

A 39-year-old lady is being induced for post dates. Her blood pressure was found to be elevated in the last few weeks of pregnancy with no significant proteinuria. She is complaining of palpitations and breathlessness. Her pulse is 98 beats/minute, and her blood pressure is found to be 130/70 mmHg. What is the most appropriate initial investigation?

L   Pulmonary embolism should be suspected, and arterial blood gas analysis will indicate hypoxia and acidosis.

Section 5: Antenatal care

36 **Antenatal screening**

37 **Genetics**

38 **Large for dates**

QUESTIONS

36 Antenatal screening

A Edwards' syndrome
B Patau's syndrome
C triploidy
D intrauterine growth restriction
E fetal death
F Noonan's syndrome
G Turner's syndrome
H neural tube defect
I Down's syndrome
J none of the above

For each description below, choose the **single** most appropriate answer from the above list of options. Each option may be used once, more than once, or not at all.

1 A patient presented to the clinic having had antenatal screening. The results of this screening were an increased nuchal translucency (3.2 mm), an alfafetoprotein (AFP) of 0.53 Multiples of Median (MoM), an unconjugated estriol (uE3) of 0.56 MoM, and an increased human chorionic gonadotrophin (hCG) of 2.6 MoM.

2 A 37-year-old lady presents to discuss the results of her antenatal screening test. The nuchal translucency is 3 mm (increased), the AFP 0.4 MoM, the uE3 0.5 MoM and the hCG 0.4 MoM.

3 A 29-year-old lady presents at 15 weeks after her triple test results. The ultrasound shows a snowstorm pattern of the placenta. The results of the triple test show that the AFP is 1.6 MoM, the hCG is 0.25 MoM and the uE3 is 0.15 MoM.

4 A 23-year-old lady presents at 20 weeks' gestation for her anomaly scan. She had a dating scan at 8 weeks' gestation that confirmed her dates. The 20-week ultrasound shows that all measurements of fetal biometry are well below the fifth centile.

Answers: see page 76.

37 Genetics

A 1:2
B 1:25
C 1:125
D Approximately 1:500
E Approximately 1:650
F 1:4
G Approximately 1:1000
H 2:3
I 1:176
J 1:220
K Approximately 1:880
L Approximately 1:1760

For each description below, choose the **single** most appropriate answer from the above list of options. Each option may be used once, more than once, or not at all.

1 The carrier risk of cystic fibrosis in Northern Europe.

2 If both the mother and her partner are carriers of cystic fibrosis, what is the risk of an affected baby?

3 If the mother is a carrier and the partner has been screened and demonstrates none of the common mutations, what is the risk of the fetus being affected?

4 What is the risk of the mother being a carrier for cystic fibrosis if her sister is affected?

Answers: see page 76.

38 Large for dates

A multiple pregnancy
B gestational diabetes mellitus
C fetal macrosomia
D fibroid uterus with red degeneration
E an adnexal mass complicating pregnancy
F gestational trophoblastic disease
G abruption with concealed haemorrhage
H a cervical fibroid
I multiple uterine fibroids
J obesity
K full bladder
L fetal hydrops
M diabetes complicating pregnancy
N wrong dates
O polyhydramnios

Choose an appropriate option for each question from the list given above.

1   A 28-year-old presents in her first pregnancy at 16 weeks' gestation with severe hyperemesis. Her blood pressure is 150/96 mmHg with 3+ of proteinuria. Her booking blood pressure is noted to be 110/70 mmHg. Abdominal examination demonstrates that the symphysis–fundus height is equivalent to 22 cm.

2   A 35-year-old presents in her second pregnancy with a new partner. She has required treatment for subfertility with one cycle of clomiphene. The gestational age calculated for the date of her last menstrual period is 18 weeks. On clinical examination of the abdomen, the symphysis–fundus height measures 26 cm.

3   A lady with insulin-dependent diabetes attends the clinic at 30 weeks of gestation. Her blood glucose monitoring reveals poor control over the past 4 weeks. On clinical examination the symphysis–fundus height measures 35 cm. Clinically, the fetal parts are difficult to determine the fetal lie and presentation.

4   An Afro-Caribbean lady presents with abdominal pain at 26 weeks of gestation. Clinical examination reveals the symphysis–fundus height as measuring 31 cm. Abdominal palpation reveals one discrete area of tenderness on the anterior wall of the uterus.

Answers: see page 77.

ANSWERS

36 Antenatal screening

Answers: I A C D

A patient presented to the clinic having had antenatal screening. The results of this screening were an increased nuchal translucency (3.2 mm), an alfafetoprotein (AFP) of 0.53 Multiples of Median (MoM), an unconjugated estriol (uE3) of 0.56 MoM, and an increased human chorionic gonadotrophin (hCG) of 2.6 MoM.

I   The combination of increased nuchal translucency and hCG with decreased AFP and uE3 is strongly suggestive of Down's syndrome.

A 37-year-old lady presents to discuss the results of her antenatal screening test. The nuchal translucency is 3 mm (increased), the AFP 0.4 MoM, the uE3 0.5 MoM and the hCG 0.4 MoM.

A   Maternal age more than 35 years, raised nuchal translucency and reduced serum markers suggest a possibility of trisomy 18.

A 29-year-old lady presents at 15 weeks after her triple test results. The ultrasound shows a snowstorm pattern of the placenta. The results of the triple test show that the AFP is 1.6 MoM, the hCG is 0.25 MoM and the uE3 is 0.15 MoM.

C   Molar changes in the presence of an associated fetus are suggestive of a partial mole. This is often due to triploidy.

A 23-year-old lady presents at 20 weeks' gestation for her anomaly scan. She had a dating scan at 8 weeks' gestation that confirmed her dates. The 20-week ultrasound shows that all measurements of fetal biometry are well below the fifth centile.

D   Early-onset intrauterine growth retardation is associated with symmetrical growth restriction and may be due to intrauterine infections or genetic causes.

37 Genetics

Answers: B F L H

The carrier risk of cystic fibrosis in Northern Europe.
B   The gene frequency in Northern Europe is 1:25.

If both the mother and her partner are carriers of cystic fibrosis, what is the risk of an affected baby?
F   The risk of inheriting an autosomal recessive disorder when both patients are carriers is 1:4.

If the mother is a carrier and the partner has been screened and demonstrates none of the common mutations, what is the risk of the fetus being affected?
L   This is equivalent to understanding that there are two alleles and that the screening tests will detect approximately 90 per cent of mutations. Therefore the risk of the baby being affected is $1:2 \times 1:2 \times 1:250 \times 1:2$.

What is the risk of the mother being a carrier for cystic fibrosis if her sister is affected?

H   An unaffected sibling of an affected person has a 2:3 chance of being a carrier.

38 Large for dates

Answers: F A O D

A 28-year-old presents in her first pregnancy at 16 weeks' gestation with severe hyperemesis. Her blood pressure is 150/96 mmHg with 3+ of proteinuria. Her booking blood pressure is noted to be 110/70 mmHg. Abdominal examination demonstrates that the symphysis–fundus height is equivalent to 22 cm.

F   Prolonged hyperemesis and early onset of pregnancy-induced hypertension suggests gestational trophoblastic disease.

A 35-year-old presents in her second pregnancy with a new partner. She has required treatment for subfertility with one cycle of clomiphene. The gestational age calculated for the date of her last menstrual period is 18 weeks. On clinical examination of the abdomen, the symphysis–fundus height measures 26 cm.

A   Ovulation induction suggests a multiple pregnancy.

A lady with insulin-dependent diabetes attends the clinic at 30 weeks of gestation. Her blood glucose monitoring reveals poor control over the past 4 weeks. On clinical examination the symphysis–fundus height measures 35 cm. Clinically, the fetal parts are difficult to determine the fetal lie and presentation.

O   Polyhydramnios is a known complication of uncontrolled diabetes mellitus.

An Afro-Caribbean lady presents with abdominal pain at 26 weeks of gestation. Clinical examination reveals the symphysis–fundus height as measuring 31 cm. Abdominal palpation reveals one discrete area of tenderness on the anterior wall of the uterus.

D   Red degeneration of a fibroid, although more common in the puerperium, can present in the antenatal period.

Section 6: Benign gynaecological conditions

39 Vulval ulcers

40 Management of fibroids

41 Uterovaginal prolapse

42 Müllerian defects

43 Management of menorrhagia

44 Cervical screening

45 Gestational trophoblastic disease

46 Paediatric gynaecology

QUESTIONS

39 Vulval ulcers

A vulval vestibulitis
B vulval squamous cell carcinoma
C lichen sclerosus
D chancroid
E lichen planus
F primary syphilis
G herpes genitalis
H scabies
I traumatic ulcer
J Beçhet's syndrome
K basal cell carcinoma
L vulval intraepithelial neoplasia
M lymphogranuloma venereum
N malignant melanoma
O vulval atrophy

For each description below, choose the **single** most appropriate answer from the above list of options. Each option may be used once, more than once, or not at all.

1   A 26-year-old woman attends the gynaecology clinic with a single, painless ulcer on her vulva. There is no associated itching. On examination there is a shallow ulcer on the right labia majora with enlarged but painless regional lymph nodes.

2   A 37-year-old lady attends the clinic with a painless vulval ulcer of 4 days' duration. She noted a papule initially, which later developed into an ulcer. She has just returned from a Caribbean holiday. Bilateral inguinal lymphadenopathy is noticed.

3   A 28-year-old lady is admitted to the surgical ward for acute urinary retention. She is already on oral antibiotics. Two days later she develops severe pain in the vulva. On examination multiple painful shallow ulcers were noted on the labia majora.

4   A 34-year-old woman attends the gynaecology clinic with dyspareunia of a few months' duration. She has recently noted pain during the insertion of tampons. On examination there is an area of focal tenderness and erythema around the vestibule. No associated lymphadenopathy is noted. Initial swabs taken by her GP are negative.

Answers: see page 87.

40 Management of fibroids

A   total hysterectomy
B   myomectomy with a prior gonadotrophin-releasing hormone (GnRH) analogue
C   total abdominal hysterectomy and bilateral salpingo-oophorectomy
D   submucosal resection of the fibroid
E   vaginal hysterectomy
F   antibiotics
G   embolisation
H   GnRH analogue
I   transcervical resection of the endometrium (TCRE)
J   catheterisation and antibiotics
K   Mirena intrauterine system
L   conservative management
M   intravenous fluids and analgesics
N   ultrasound monitoring
O   GnRH analogue followed by hysterectomy

For each description below, choose the **single** most appropriate answer from the above list of options. Each option may be used once, more than once, or not at all.

1   A 45-year-old nulliparous woman is being evaluated for inflammatory bowel disease as an inpatient. Ultrasound showed a 5 cm fundal fibroid and a 3 cm anterior wall fibroid. Her periods are regular: 4–5 days in 30 days. She denies any intermenstrual bleeding. She is up to date with smears, with normal results.

2   A 36-year-old nulliparous woman is being evaluated for secondary subfertility. She has regular heavy periods lasting for 7 days every month. Ultrasound shows a 4 cm-sized pedunculated fibroid impinging into the uterine cavity.

3   A 34-year-old para 1 presents 4 weeks after her delivery with vomiting and abdominal pain. She is complaining of vaginal bleeding that started 3 days ago. Her haemoglobin level is 8.8 g/dL. On examination, the uterus is about 18-week size. There is fresh vaginal bleeding. Ultrasound shows an enlarged uterus without any retained products of conception.

4   A 43-year-old patient is admitted with acute urinary retention, fever and dysuria. She recollects having heavy periods for the past few months. On examination there is a central, 20-week-sized mass.

5   A 40-year-old Afro-Caribbean lady presents to her GP with dysmenorrhoea and heavy periods. Her haemoglobin is 9 g/dL. Ultrasound of the pelvis shows a 26-week-size uterus with multiple fibroids. What is the appropriate management?

Answers: see page 87.

41 Uterovaginal prolapse

A   vaginal hysterectomy
B   pelvic floor exercises
C   local oestrogens
D   do nothing
E   ring pessary and oestrogens
F   anterior colporrhaphy
G   posterior colporrhaphy
H   colpoclesis
I   shelf pessary
J   transvaginal sacrospinous fixation
K   laparoscopic sacrocolpopexy
L   open sacrocolpopexy
M   posterior intravaginal sling plasty
N   Fothergill repair
O   vaginal hysterectomy with pelvic floor repair

For each description below, choose the **single** most appropriate answer from the above list of options. Each option may be used once, more than once, or not at all.

1   A 62-year-old lady attends the gynaecology clinic with a mass descending per vaginum. She underwent total abdominal hysterectomy with bilateral salpingo-oophorectomy 10 years ago for severe menorrhagia. On examination there is a grade II vault prolapse with poor pelvic tone.

2   An 82-year-old lady has a complete vaginal prolapse. She is living in a nursing home and suffers from severe dementia, frequent urinary retention and ischaemic heart disease. On examination she has a grade III uterovaginal prolapse with a grade III cystocele and rectocele. There is a 2 cm decubitus ulcer on the cervix. The vaginal wall is thin and atrophic.

3   A 34-year-old para 2 attends the gynaecology clinic for difficulty during defaecation. The problem started after her second delivery and is gradually getting worse. She occasionally has to digitalise before defaecation. There are no urinary symptoms. There is no obvious cystocele or cervical descent, but she does have a grade II rectocele.

4   A 50-year-old postmenopausal woman presents with discomfort during sexual intercourse. She went through the menopause at the age of 40. She suffers from severe vaginal dryness for which she was prescribed local oestrogens 6 months ago. On examination she has a grade I cystocele and second-degree uterine prolapse.

5   A 34-year-old woman presents to the gynaecology clinic with stress incontinence. She had a forceps delivery 6 weeks ago. On examination there is no pelvic organ prolapse.

Answers: see page 88.

42 Müllerian defects

A Strassman surgery
B vaginoplasty
C observation
D psychosexual counselling
E computed tomography (CT) for renal/müllerian defects
F hysteroscopic resection
G utriculoplasty
H cruciate incision
I abdominoperineal septal resection
J hormonal replacement therapy
K removal of gonads
L karyotyping

For each description below, choose the **single** most appropriate answer from the above list of options. Each option may be used once, more than once, or not at all.

1 A 15-year-old girl is referred by her GP for primary amenorrhoea. Her secondary sexual characteristics are normal. She recollects having recent cyclical abdominal pain. Her follicle-stimulating hormone (FSH) level is 10 IU/ml, and her luteinising hormone (LH) level 11 IU/ml. The free androgen index is normal. Ultrasound of the pelvis shows a right-sided ovarian cyst of 4 cm. Vaginal examination reveals a complete transverse septum in the lower vagina. What is the next step?

2 An 11-year-old girl undergoes a laparotomy for appendicitis. On opening the abdomen there is noted to be a torted gangrenous ovarian cyst, for which she undergoes a unilateral oophorectomy. Further exploration reveals a complete absence of the uterus and both fallopian tubes. The renal tract appears normal. Vaginal examination reveals a blind pouch of 3 cm length. FSH, LH and serum oestradiol levels are normal.

3 A 20-year-old woman is being evaluated for bowel problems. Ultrasound of the pelvis and abdomen shows a bicornuate uterus. Renal tract imaging shows no abnormalities. She is not in a relationship and not planning a family in the near future.

Answers: see page 89.

43 Management of menorrhagia

A Danazol
B endometrial ablation
C transcervical resection of the endometrium
D vaginal hysterectomy
E levonorgestrel-releasing intrauterine system
F cyclical norethisterone
G tranexamic acid
H abdominal hysterectomy
I mefenamic acid
J gonadotrophin-releasing hormone analogues
K reassurance
L combined oral contraceptive pills
M total abdominal hysterectomy
N pelvic ultrasound
O hysteroscopy and endometrial biopsy
P triple swabs

For each description below, choose the **single** most appropriate answer from the above list of options. Each option may be used once, more than once, or not at all.

1 A 15-year-old girl presents 6 months after her menarche with continuous bleeding for 3 weeks on two occasions. She is not sexually active.

2 A 33-year-old para 2 lady presents with cyclical heavy bleeding. She is not contemplating a pregnancy as she has recently broken up with her partner.

3 A 47-year-old presents with irregular, heavy bleeding. She is para 2 and has been sterilised. She continues to bleed with cyclical progesterone prescribed by her GP.

4 A 26-year-old lady presents with intermenstrual bleeding during the second week of her cycle. She was investigated for the same problem in the previous year. She has no postcoital bleeding and is trying to become pregnant.

5 A 44-year-old Afro-Caribbean nulliparous lady presents with 2-year history of dysmenorrhoea and menorrhagia. She has a large central lower abdominal mass, which has been confirmed as a 20-week-size fibroid. Ultrasound has shown multiple fibroids, and her recent haemoglobin level was 84 mg/dl.

Answers: see page 90.

44 Cervical screening

A   refer to colposcopy
B   large loop excision of the transformation zone
C   colposcopy-directed cervical biopsy
D   high vaginal swab and *Chlamydia* swab
E   reassurance
F   cone biopsy – knife
G   perform a first smear test
H   await the next smear test results
I   punch biopsy of the cervix on naked-eye examination
J   Pipelle endometrial sampling
K   hysteroscopy and endometrial biopsy
L   smear test after childbirth
M   refer to colposcopy within 2 weeks

For each description below, choose the **single** most appropriate answer from the above list of options. Each option may be used once, more than once, or not at all.

1   A 28-year-old pregnant lady presents with bleeding per vaginum at 20 weeks of pregnancy. Ultrasound reveals an active appropriately grown fetus with a small area of retroplacental haematoma. The cervix appears normal on clinical examination. She has had no smear tests so far. What is appropriate management?

2   A 25-year-old lady has a routine smear and is reported as having moderate dyskaryosis. What is appropriate management?

3   A 32-year-old lady has a routine smear and is noted to have borderline endocervical cell changes. What is appropriate management?

4   A 46-year-old lady is being followed up with an annual smear for a previous abnormal smear. The smear has been reported to have possible cancerous cells. What is appropriate management?

Answers: see page 90.

45 Gestational trophoblastic disease

A intramuscular methotrexate
B evacuation and curettage
C mifepristone followed by misoprostol
D evacuation and curettage and referral to an appropriate centre
E explain the diagnosis and refer to an appropriate centre
F prostaglandin E2
G conservative treatment
H intravenous dactinomycin
I evacuation and curettage and referral to an appropriate centre with the histology results
J EMA-CO (etoposide–methotrexate–dactinomycin–cyclophosphamide–vincristine)
K termination of pregnancy

For each description below, choose the **single** most appropriate answer from the above list of options. Each option may be used once, more than once, or not at all.

1 A 20-year-old primigravida attends the emergency gynaecology department with vaginal bleeding at 14 weeks' gestation. Her ultrasound shows a snowstorm appearance. What is the most appropriate step?

2 A 28-year-old woman undergoes an emergency evacuation of retained products of conception for incomplete miscarriage at 12 weeks' gestation. Histopathological examination of the specimen shows partial trophoblastic changes. What is the most appropriate step?

3 A 29-year-old lady undergoes a nuchal translucency at 13 weeks' gestation. She is found to have a twin pregnancy with a molar pregnancy and a viable intrauterine pregnancy. What is the most appropriate step?

4 A 28-year-old lady presents 4 weeks after a normal delivery with a sudden onset of severe bleeding. She passes chunky tissue resembling placenta; this is sent for histology and is reported as trophoblastic tissues. She is seen in the referral clinic and a decision is made to initiate chemotherapy.

Answers: see page 91.

46 Paediatric gynaecology

A 21-alpha hydroxylase deficiency
B 11-beta hydroxylase deficiency
C 3-beta hydroxylase steroid dehydrogenase deficiency
D complete androgen insensitivity syndrome
E partial androgen insensitivity syndrome
F Turner's syndrome
G müllerian agenesis
H mixed gonadal dysgenesis
I panhypopituitarism
J Kallman's syndrome
K Beckwith–Weidemann syndrome
L Rokitansky–Kuster–Hauser syndrome
M Laron's syndrome
N Turner's mosaic

For each description below, choose the **single** most appropriate answer from the above list of options. Each option may be used once, more than once, or not at all.

1 A 16-year-old presents to the clinic with primary amenorrhoea. She has otherwise been well. She has no pelvic or axillary hair but her breasts are well developed. Ultrasound examination shows complete absence of the uterus.

2 A 2-day-old child on the postnatal ward is referred for ambiguous genitalia. On examination the child has a small phallus and bifid scrotum with palpable testes. No female structures are visible on a pelvic ultrasound. Karyotyping is 46XY. Blood pressure and serum electrolytes are normal. Plasma testosterone levels are elevated.

3 A 5-day-old child is seen with ambiguous genitalia. There is a small phallus and what appears to be the labioscrotal folds are partially fused. No testes are palpable. The blood pressure is found to be elevated.

4 A 16-year-old girl presents with primary amenorrhoea. Her breast development is Tanner stage 2. Pubic and axillary hair show stage I development. The girl appears otherwise well. Ultrasound shows the presence of a normal uterus and tubes. Her height is 140 cm.

Answers: see page 91.

ANSWERS

39 Vulval ulcers

Answers: F D G A

A 26-year-old woman attends the gynaecology clinic with a single, painless ulcer on her vulva. There is no associated itching. On examination there is a shallow ulcer on the right labia majora with enlarged but painless regional lymph nodes.

F   Primary syphilis presents with shallow, punched-out ulcers with or without associated lymphadenopathy about 10–90 days following initial exposure.

A 37-year-old lady attends the clinic with a painless vulval ulcer of 4 days' duration. She noted a papule initially, which later developed into an ulcer. She has just returned from a Caribbean holiday. Bilateral inguinal lymphadenopathy is noticed.

D   The history is characteristic of chancroid caused by *Haemophilus ducreyi*, a Gram-negative streptobacillus.

A 28-year-old lady is admitted to the surgical ward for acute urinary retention. She is already on oral antibiotics. Two days later she develops severe pain in the vulva. On examination multiple painful shallow ulcers were noted on the labia majora.

G   Urinary retention often precedes the development of genital herpes.

A 34-year-old woman attends the gynaecology clinic with dyspareunia of a few months' duration. She has recently noted pain during the insertion of tampons. On examination there is an area of focal tenderness and erythema around the vestibule. No associated lymphadenopathy is noted. Initial swabs taken by her GP are negative.

A   Vulval vestibulitis often presents with tenderness alone. Infection screening is negative, and infections are difficult to treat.

40 Management of fibroids

Answers: L D M J O

A 45-year-old nulliparous woman is being evaluated for inflammatory bowel disease as an inpatient. Ultrasound showed a 5 cm fundal fibroid and a 3 cm anterior wall fibroid. Her periods are regular: 4–5 days in 30 days. She denies any intermenstrual bleeding. She is up to date with smears, with normal results.

L   Incidental finding of a fibroid occurs in up to 30 per cent of women in the reproductive age group. No intervention is required if the fibroid is asymptomatic.

A 36-year-old nulliparous woman is being evaluated for secondary subfertility. She has regular heavy periods lasting for 7 days every month. Ultrasound shows a 4 cm-sized pedunculated fibroid impinging into the uterine cavity.

D Subfertility can be caused by a submucosal fibroid acting as an intrauterine contraceptive device. If other factors are normal, submucosal resection is often considered.

A 34-year-old para 1 presents 4 weeks after her delivery with vomiting and abdominal pain. She is complaining of vaginal bleeding that started 3 days ago. Her haemoglobin level is 8.8 g/dL. On examination, the uterus is about 18-week size. There is fresh vaginal bleeding. Ultrasound shows an enlarged uterus without any retained products of conception.
M Red degeneration of a fibroid commonly occurs in the postpartum period. Hydration and adequate analgesia are the first-line management.

A 43-year-old patient is admitted with acute urinary retention, fever and dysuria. She recollects having heavy periods for the past few months. On examination there is a central, 20-week-sized mass.
J Large fibroids cause impaction of the uterus and lead to urinary retention. Obstruction with residual urine could lead to recurrent urinary tract infection.

A 40-year-old Afro-Caribbean lady presents to her GP with dysmenorrhoea and heavy periods. Her haemoglobin is 9 g/dL. Ultrasound of the pelvis shows a 26-week-size uterus with multiple fibroids. What is the appropriate management?
O Fibroids causing menorrhagia leading to anaemia are often resistant to conservative measures. Hysterectomy is often required. Prior treatment with GnRH helps to reduce bleeding and decrease the size of the fibroid.

41 Uterovaginal prolapse

Answers: L E G O B

A 62-year-old lady attends the gynaecology clinic with a mass descending per vaginum. She underwent total abdominal hysterectomy with bilateral salpingo-oophorectomy 10 years ago for severe menorrhagia. On examination there is a grade II vault prolapse with poor pelvic tone.
L Open/abdominal sacrocolpopexy is appropriate for vault prolapse. Up to 93 per cent success has been reported.

An 82-year-old lady has a complete vaginal prolapse. She is living in a nursing home and suffers from severe dementia, frequent urinary retention and ischaemic heart disease. On examination she has a grade III uterovaginal prolapse with a grade III cystocele and rectocele. There is a 2 cm decubitus ulcer on the cervix. The vaginal wall is thin and atrophic.
E Ring pessaries are designed to provide support to the uterus and upper vagina. The use of local oestrogens and initial packing promotes the healing of a decubitus ulcer. This patient is not suitable for surgery, and a conservative approach would be more appropriate.

A 34-year-old para 2 attends the gynaecology clinic for difficulty during defaecation. The problem started after her second delivery and is gradually getting

worse. She occasionally has to digitalise before defaecation. There are no urinary symptoms. There is no obvious cystocele or cervical descent, but she does have a grade II rectocele.

G   Isolated posterior compartment defects often result from childbirth. Correction of the defect in the rectovaginal septum and deficient perineum will improve defaecatory function.

A 50-year-old postmenopausal woman presents with discomfort during sexual intercourse. She went through the menopause at the age of 40. She suffers from severe vaginal dryness for which she was prescribed local oestrogens 6 months ago. On examination she has a grade I cystocele and second-degree uterine prolapse.

O   Vaginal hysterectomy with pelvic floor repair is the treatment of choice in symptomatic prolapse after menopause.

A 34-year-old woman presents to the gynaecology clinic with stress incontinence. She had a forceps delivery 6 weeks ago. On examination there is no pelvic organ prolapse.

B   Pelvic floor exercises are particularly useful in woman up to 6 months following vaginal delivery.

42 Müllerian defects

Answers: I B C

A 15-year-old girl is referred by her GP for primary amenorrhoea. Her secondary sexual characteristics are normal. She recollects having recent cyclical abdominal pain. Her follicle-stimulating hormone (FSH) level is 10 IU/ml, and her luteinising hormone (LH) level 11 IU/ml. The free androgen index is normal. Ultrasound of the pelvis shows a right-sided ovarian cyst of 4 cm. Vaginal examination reveals a complete transverse septum in the lower vagina. What is the next step?

I   A transverse vaginal septum requires complete removal by an abdominoperineal approach to prevent post-surgical stenosis. Childhood vaginal enlargement surgery may require revision in up to 90 per cent of cases.

An 11-year-old girl undergoes a laparotomy for appendicitis. On opening the abdomen there is noted to be a torted gangrenous ovarian cyst, for which she undergoes a unilateral oophorectomy. Further exploration reveals a complete absence of the uterus and both fallopian tubes. The renal tract appears normal. Vaginal examination reveals a blind pouch of 3 cm length. FSH, LH and serum oestradiol levels are normal.

B   Complete müllerian agenesis leads to a complete absence of the tubes and uterus. Vaginoplasty after detailed counselling could preserve sexual function.

A 20-year-old woman is being evaluated for bowel problems. Ultrasound of the pelvis and abdomen shows a bicornuate uterus. Renal tract imaging shows no abnormalities. She is not in a relationship and not planning a family in the near future.

C   Incidental uterine anomalies need not be treated. However, detailed counselling regarding pregnancy outcome is necessary.

BENIGN GYNAECOLOGICAL CONDITIONS

43 Management of menorrhagia

Answers: L E O P M

A 15-year-old girl presents 6 months after her menarche with continuous bleeding for 3 weeks on two occasions. She is not sexually active.

L   The most likely diagnosis is anovulatory bleeding, which is common in teenage girls (55 per cent of cycles are anovulatory in the first year following menarche). The combined oral contraceptive pill is ideal even if they are not sexually active.

A 33-year-old para 2 lady presents with cyclical heavy bleeding. She is not contemplating a pregnancy as she has recently broken up with her partner.

E   A Mirena intrauterine system is a good choice for a parous woman also needing contraception.

A 47-year-old presents with irregular, heavy bleeding. She is para 2 and has been sterilised. She continues to bleed with cyclical progesterone prescribed by her GP.

O   Perimenopausal irregular bleeding should be assessed by hysteroscopy and endometrial biopsy.

A 26-year-old lady presents with intermenstrual bleeding during the second week of her cycle. She was investigated for the same problem in the previous year. She has no postcoital bleeding and is trying to become pregnant.

P   Pelvic infection (*Chlamydia*) is the likely cause of intermenstrual bleeding in this age group of 15–30-year-olds.

A 44-year-old Afro-Caribbean nulliparous lady presents with 2-year history of dysmenorrhoea and menorrhagia. She has a large central lower abdominal mass, which has been confirmed as a 20-week-size fibroid. Ultrasound has shown multiple fibroids, and her recent haemoglobin level was 84 mg/dl.

M   Both hysterectomy and uterine artery embolisation can be considered with large fibroids.

44 Cervical screening

Answers: L A A M

A 28-year-old pregnant lady presents with bleeding per vaginum at 20 weeks of pregnancy. Ultrasound reveals an active appropriately grown fetus with a small area of retroplacental haematoma. The cervix appears normal on clinical examination. She has had no smear tests so far. What is appropriate management?

L   Smear tests are generally not advised during pregnancy, especially if the cervix looks normal. A conservative approach is adopted.

A 25-year-old lady has a routine smear and is reported as having moderate dyskaryosis. What is appropriate management?

A   Cervical intraepithelial neoplasia I must ideally be referred for colposcopy.

A 32-year-old lady has a routine smear and is noted to have borderline endocervical cell changes. What is appropriate management?

A   Borderline endocervical cells must be referred immediately for colposcopy.

A 46-year-old lady is being followed up with an annual smear for a previous abnormal smear. The smear has been reported to have possible cancerous cells. What is appropriate management?

M   Suspected invasive cancer must be referred under the 2-week rule.

45 Gestational trophoblastic disease

Answers: I E G J

A 20-year-old primigravida attends the emergency gynaecology department with vaginal bleeding at 14 weeks' gestation. Her ultrasound shows a snowstorm appearance. What is the most appropriate step?

I   Confirmation of histology is essential before referring the patient to the referral centre.

A 28-year-old woman undergoes an emergency evacuation of retained products of conception for incomplete miscarriage at 12 weeks' gestation. Histopathological examination of the specimen shows partial trophoblastic changes. What is the most appropriate step?

E   Patients with a molar pregnancy should receive adequate counselling regarding follow-up.

A 29-year-old lady undergoes a nuchal translucency at 13 weeks' gestation. She is found to have a twin pregnancy with a molar pregnancy and a viable intrauterine pregnancy. What is the most appropriate step?

G   Successful pregnancy outcome occurs in a third of cases. Persistent trophoblastic disease requiring chemotherapy is more frequent in twin pregnancy.

A 28-year-old lady presents 4 weeks after a normal delivery with a sudden onset of severe bleeding. She passes chunky tissue resembling placenta; this is sent for histology and is reported as trophoblastic tissues. She is seen in the referral clinic and a decision is made to initiate chemotherapy.

J   Postpartum presentation is a high risk factor, and the EMA-CO regimen would be appropriate.

46 Paediatric gynaecology

Answers: D E B F

A 16-year-old presents to the clinic with primary amenorrhoea. She has otherwise been well. She has no pelvic or axillary hair but her breasts are well developed. Ultrasound examination shows complete absence of the uterus.

D   Complete androgen insensitivity syndrome, previously known as testicular feminising syndrome, is characterised by müllerian structures, normal female genitalia and absent pubic hair with high levels of circulating testosterone.

BENIGN GYNAECOLOGICAL CONDITIONS

A 2-day-old child on the postnatal ward is referred for ambiguous genitalia. On examination the child has a small phallus and bifid scrotum with palpable testes. No female structures are visible on a pelvic ultrasound. Karyotyping is 46XY. Blood pressure and serum electrolytes are normal. Plasma testosterone levels are elevated.

E   Partial androgen insensitivity syndrome can present with ambiguous genitalia.

A 5-day-old child is seen with ambiguous genitalia. There is a small phallus and what appears to be the labioscrotal folds are partially fused. No testes are palpable. The blood pressure is found to be elevated.

B   11-Beta-hydroxylase is the second most common variant of congenital adrenal hyperplasia and accounts for approximately 5 per cent of cases. It presents with features of androgen excess, including the masculinisation of female newborns and precocious puberty in male children. Approximately two-thirds of cases also have hypertension.

A 16-year-old girl presents with primary amenorrhoea. Her breast development is Tanner stage 2. Pubic and axillary hair show stage I development. The girl appears otherwise well. Ultrasound shows the presence of a normal uterus and tubes. Her height is 140 cm.

F   Turner's syndrome can present as primary amenorrhoea. Turner's mosaic can present with secondary amenorrhoea.

Section 7: Gynaecological oncology

47 Management of endometrial cancer

48 Treatment of cervical cancer

49 Vulval carcinoma

50 Management of adnexal mass

51 Colposcopy

QUESTIONS

47 Management of endometrial cancer

A laparotomy and bilateral salpingo-oophorectomy (BSO)
B laparoscopically assisted vaginal hysterectomy
C radical hysterectomy, radiotherapy and chemotherapy
D external radiotherapy
E presurgical radiotherapy followed by completion hysterectomy
F chemoradiation
G palliative care
H total abdominal hysterectomy (TAH) with BSO, peritoneal cytology and selective lymphadenectomy
I tamoxifen
J progesterone
K TAH, BSO, peritoneal cytology, omectectomy ± pelvic para-aortic lymphadenectomy.
L laparoscopic bilateral salpingectomy
M annual follow-up
N optimal debulking surgery
O combined surgery and chemotherapy

For each description below, choose the **single** most appropriate answer from the above list of options. Each option may be used once, more than once, or not at all.

1 A 38-year-old parous woman underwent simple hysterectomy with ovarian conservation for severe menorrhagia. Later histopathological examination has shown a well-differentiated endometrial adenocarcinoma limited to the endometrium. What is the appropriate next step?

2 A 51-year-old lady undergoes outpatient hysteroscopy and endometrial sampling for postmenopausal bleeding. Histopathological examination has shown well-differentiated adenocarcinoma cells. A subsequent magnetic resonance imaging (MRI) scan has shown a right lateral uterine wall growth limited to the inner one third of the myometrium. The uterus is found to be of normal size. What is the next step?

3 A 50-year-old nulliparous woman was referred to the gynaecology clinic with irregular vaginal bleeding and abdominal pain lasting 2 months. She has also noted some abdominal distension. Pelvic ultrasound showed an enlarged uterus with 14 mm thick endometrium and a 10 cm complex adnexal mass on the right side. Outpatient Pipelle sampling has shown well-differentiated endometroid adeno-carcinoma cells. Subsequent MRI has shown a three-quarters myometrial invasion. What is the most appropriate option?

4 A 37-year-old lady has been seen in the gynaecology clinic with irregular vaginal bleeding for the past 2 months. She has previously been diagnosed with breast

cancer and has been on tamoxifen for 14 years. Pelvic ultrasound and outpatient hysteroscopy are normal. Histology of the endometrial sample has shown atypical endometrial hyperplasia.

5 A 58-year-old lady has been seen with postmenopausal bleeding lasting for 2 months. She has noted recent abdominal distension. Pelvic ultrasound has shown a growth involving the uterine wall, with normal adnexa. There is free fluid in the abdomen. MRI scanning shows full-thickness myometrial invasion. Histology of the endometrial sample obtained shows uterine papillary serous adenocarcinoma cells with poor differentiation.

Answers: see page 100.

48 Treatment of cervical cancer

A interstitial radiotherapy
B radical hysterectomy and pelvic lymphadenectomy
C large loop excision of the transformation zone (LLETZ)
D simple hysterectomy
E chemotherapy
F no further treatment
G intracavitary radiotherapy
H laparoscopic lymphadenectomy
I trachelectomy
J chemotherapy external beam radiotherapy and brachytherapy
K palliative multidisciplinary care
L cone biopsy of the cervix
M annual smear examinations
N subtotal hysterectomy
O pelvic exenteration

For each description below, choose the **single** most appropriate answer from the above list of options. Each option may be used once, more than once, or not at all.

1   A 32-year-old nulliparous lady has a smear showing possible cancer cells. Subsequent colposcopy, biopsy, examination under anaesthesia (EUA), magnetic resonance imaging (MRI) and cystoscopy show a lesion confined to the cervix with a maximum dimension of 3 cm. She has been trying for a pregnancy for the past 6 months. What is the most appropriate option?

2   A 32-year-old nulliparous lady has cancer cells found on a routine smear. Subsequent colposcopy, biopsy, EUA, MRI and cystoscopy show a lesion confined to the cervix with a maximum dimension of 6 × 4.8 cm. She has been trying for a pregnancy for the past 6 months. What is the most appropriate treatment option?

3   A 42-year-old multiparous woman who has never had a smear presents with post-coital bleeding and is found to have cervical carcinoma extending to the parametrium with left-sided hydronephrosis. What is the most appropriate option?

4   A 52-year-old lady was referred to colposcopy with severe dyskaryosis. Colposcopy showed changes consistent with cervical intraepithelial neoplasia (CIN) III. LLETZ was performed. Histopathology reported a cervical tumour to a depth of 2 mm and a maximal horizontal spread of 5 mm. Excisional margins were clear of the disease. What is an appropriate option?

5   A 58-year-old Asian lady who has never previously had a smear presents with postmenopausal bleeding. Investigations show a bulky cervical cancer with extension to the bladder mucosa and spread confined to the liver capsule. What is an appropriate option?

Answers: see page 101.

49 Vulval carcinoma

A radical vulvectomy
B local oestrogen cream
C laser coagulation
D targeted multiple punch biopsies
E 5-flurouracil cream
F simple vulvectomy
G wide local excision and bilateral groin node dissection
H preoperative radiotherapy
I immunotherapy
J wide local excision with sentinel node dissection
K wide local excision with ipsilateral groin node dissection
L steroid cream
M conjugated equine oestrogens and progestogens
N chemotherapy
O wide local excision with a 1 cm margin

For each description below, choose the **single** most appropriate answer from the above list of options. Each option may be used once, more than once, or not at all.

1 A 53-year-old postmenopausal woman presented to her GP with vulval itching and soreness. On examination she had a 1.5 cm raised lesion on her right labia majora, which was biopsied. Histology has shown an invasive squamous cell carcinoma with stromal invasion less than 1 mm. What is an appropriate option?

2 A 76-year-old woman presents with vulval itching and bleeding. She suffers from mild dementia and has been treated in the past for vulval dystrophy. On examination there is a 4 cm ulcerating lesion fixed to pubic bone on left labia majora with palpable nodes on the right side. A biopsy confirms squamous cell carcinoma. What is an appropriate option?

3 A 69-year-old lady is seen in the gynaecology outpatient clinic with vulval soreness and itching. On examination she has a 15 mm lesion on the right labia minora close to the fourchette. The distance from the edge of the lesion and the midline is about 1.5 cm, with no palpable nodes. Histology shows squamous cell carcinoma. What is an appropriate option?

4 A 56-year-old postmenopausal woman presents with a history of vulval itching and soreness of a few years' duration. On examination the vulva appears dry with scaly lesions throughout. Subsequent biopsy shows epithelial thinning and inflammatory changes suggesting lichen sclerosus. What is an appropriate option?

Answers: see page 101.

50 Management of adnexal mass

A   radiotherapy
B   do nothing
C   laparoscopic cystectomy
D   CA 125
E   computed tomography (CT) of the abdomen and pelvis
F   repeat ultrasound in 4–6 months
G   ultrasound-guided cyst aspiration
H   laparoscopic bilateral oophorectomy
I   discharge from follow-up
J   diagnostic laparoscopy
K   laparotomy, total abdominal hysterectomy and bilateral salpingo-oophorectomy
L   neoadjuvant chemotherapy
M   laparotomy and removal of cyst
N   second-look laparotomy
O   optimal debulking

For each description below, choose the **single** most appropriate answer from the above list of options. Each option may be used once, more than once, or not at all.

1   An 18-year-old girl presents with urinary frequency. On examination she is found to have a lower abdominal mass. Ultrasound shows a 7 cm left-sided ovarian mass with mixed echogenicity. CT confirms the findings with fatty contents in the cyst, but no other pathology is seen. CA 125 and carcinoembryonic antigen levels are normal. What is an appropriate management option?

2   A 47-year-old perimenopausal lady had a pelvic scan for menorrhagia and was found to have a 4 cm anechoic thin-walled cyst. The CA 125 level is 18 units/mL. What is an appropriate management option?

3   A 54-year-old postmenopausal woman presents with an asymptomatic 4 cm ovarian cyst, which has persisted for a year. CA 125 level is normal. What is an appropriate management option?

4   A 32-year-old anxious lady presents with lower abdominal pain. She has a past history of irritable bowel syndrome. Pelvic ultrasound showed a 4 cm ovarian cyst, which was followed up 6 months later, when the cyst was reported to be 5 cm. Serum CA 125 was normal on both occasions. What is an appropriate management option?

Answers: see page 102.

51 Colposcopy

A colposcopy-directed biopsy
B total abdominal hysterectomy
C excision of the abnormal area
D large loop excision of the transformation zone (LLETZ)
E elective radiotherapy
F chemotherapy
G chemoradiation
H trachelectomy
I Wertheim's hysterectomy
J vaginal hysterectomy
K Schauta-Mitra's hysterectomy
L radical hysterectomy and pelvic lymphadenectomy
M palliative radiotherapy
N emergency radiotherapy
O packing with Monsel's solution

For each description below, choose the **single** most appropriate answer from the above list of options. Each option may be used once, more than once, or not at all.

1 A 26-year-old lady is referred for colposcopy with mild dyskaryosis. Colposcopic examination suggests two areas of cervical intraepithelial neoplasia (CIN) I changes. What is appropriate management?

2 A 50-year-old lady is referred with moderate dyskaryosis and is diagnosed with CIN II on colposcopy. What is appropriate management?

3 A 54-year-old Asian lady who has never had a smear presents with heavy bleeding and has a suspicious ulcerative lesion on her cervix. Further investigations reveal a stage III B cervical cancer.

4 A 36-year-old lady is referred to colposcopy with severe dyskaryosis. On examination there are three acetowhite areas without uptake of iodine, suggestive of CIN III.

5 A 45-year-old lady with known stage III cervical carcinoma presents with acute onset of heavy bleeding. She has bled through the vaginal pack. She is haemodynamically stable after an estimated 700 mL blood loss.

Answers: see page 103.

ANSWERS

47 Management of endometrial cancer

Answers: A H K G C

A 38-year-old parous woman underwent simple hysterectomy with ovarian conservation for severe menorrhagia. Later histopathological examination has shown a well-differentiated endometrial adenocarcinoma limited to the endometrium. What is the appropriate next step?

A   TAH with BSO is adequate for stage Ia disease. BSO may be performed by laparotomy.

A 51-year-old lady undergoes outpatient hysteroscopy and endometrial sampling for postmenopausal bleeding. Histopathological examination has shown well-differentiated adenocarcinoma cells. A subsequent magnetic resonance imaging (MRI) scan has shown a right lateral uterine wall growth limited to the inner one third of the myometrium. The uterus is found to be of normal size. What is the next step?

H   TAH, BSO, peritoneal cytology ± pelvic para-aortic lymphadenectomy is the standard procedure for stage Ib disease.

A 50-year-old nulliparous woman was referred to the gynaecology clinic with irregular vaginal bleeding and abdominal pain lasting 2 months. She has also noted some abdominal distension. Pelvic ultrasound showed an enlarged uterus with 14 mm thick endometrium and a 10 cm complex adnexal mass on the right side. Outpatient Pipelle sampling has shown well-differentiated endometroid adenocarcinoma cells. Subsequent MRI has shown a three-quarters myometrial invasion. What is the most appropriate option?

K   Primary site (ovary or endometrium) is difficult to define in endometroid cell differentiation. Laparotomy may show more clues to ovarian pathology.

A 37-year-old lady has been seen in the gynaecology clinic with irregular vaginal bleeding for the past 2 months. She has previously been diagnosed with breast cancer and has been on tamoxifen for 14 years. Pelvic ultrasound and outpatient hysteroscopy are normal. Histology of the endometrial sample has shown atypical endometrial hyperplasia.

G   TAH and BSO will be adequate treatment for atypical hyperplasia. A detailed histopathological examination should be undertaken for concomitant endometrial carcinoma.

A 58-year-old lady has been seen with postmenopausal bleeding lasting for 2 months. She has noted recent abdominal distension. Pelvic ultrasound has shown a growth involving the uterine wall, with normal adnexa. There is free fluid in the abdomen. MRI scanning shows full-thickness myometrial invasion. Histology of the endometrial sample obtained shows uterine papillary serous adenocarcinoma cells with poor differentiation.

C   Both uterine papillary serous adenocarcinoma and clear cell carcinoma are aggressive tumours, requiring radiotherapy and chemotherapy.

48 Treatment of cervical cancer

Answers: I B J M K

A 32-year-old nulliparous lady has a smear showing possible cancer cells. Subsequent colposcopy, biopsy, examination under anaesthesia (EUA), magnetic resonance imaging (MRI) and cystoscopy show a lesion confined to the cervix with a maximum dimension of 3 cm. She has been trying for a pregnancy for the past 6 months. What is the most appropriate option?

I   In stage Ib1 disease, trachelectomy would be an option for disease measuring less than 4 cm in women wishing to retain their fertility.

A 32-year-old nulliparous lady has cancer cells found on a routine smear. Subsequent colposcopy, biopsy, EUA, MRI and cystoscopy show a lesion confined to the cervix with a maximum dimension of 6 × 4.8 cm. She has been trying for a pregnancy for the past 6 months. What is the most appropriate treatment option?

B   For stage Ib2 disease, large-volume disease (>4 cm), both radical surgery and radiotherapy could be considered. Trachelectomy is not an option beyond stage Ib1. Surgery is preferred to radiotherapy in young women.

A 42-year-old multiparous woman who has never had a smear presents with post-coital bleeding and is found to have cervical carcinoma extending to the para-metrium with left-sided hydronephrosis. What is the most appropriate option?

J   Stage IIIb disease needs combined radiotherapy and chemotherapy.

A 52-year-old lady was referred to colposcopy with severe dyskaryosis. Colposcopy showed changes consistent with cervical intraepithelial neoplasia (CIN) III. LLETZ was performed. Histopathology reported a cervical tumour to a depth of 2 mm and a maximal horizontal spread of 5 mm. Excisional margins were clear of the disease. What is an appropriate option?

M   If the LLETZ margins are clear, no further treatment is required, but follow-up with smears is needed. This is consistent with stage Ia1 tumour – a horizontal spread of 7 mm and a depth of 5 mm.

A 58-year-old Asian lady who has never previously had a smear presents with postmenopausal bleeding. Investigations show a bulky cervical cancer with extension to the bladder mucosa and spread confined to the liver capsule. What is an appropriate option?

K   Stage IVb disease needs individualised multidisciplinary palliative approach.

49 Vulval carcinoma

Answers: O H G L

A 53-year-old postmenopausal woman presented to her GP with vulval itching and soreness. On examination she had a 1.5 cm raised lesion on her right labia majora, which was biopsied. Histology has shown an invasive squamous cell carcinoma with stromal invasion less than 1 mm. What is an appropriate option?

O   Wide local excision to achieve a 1 cm disease-free margin is a recommended option for stage Ia disease.

A 76-year-old woman presents with vulval itching and bleeding. She suffers from mild dementia and has been treated in the past for vulval dystrophy. On examination there is a 4 cm ulcerating lesion fixed to pubic bone on left labia majora with palpable nodes on the right side. A biopsy confirms squamous cell carcinoma. What is an appropriate option?

H   Preoperative radiotherapy and neoadjuvant chemotherapy are helpful to shrink the tumour prior to surgery.

A 69-year-old lady is seen in the gynaecology outpatient clinic with vulval soreness and itching. On examination she has a 15 mm lesion on the right labia minora close to the fourchette. The distance from the edge of the lesion and the midline is about 1.5 cm, with no palpable nodes. Histology shows squamous cell carcinoma. What is an appropriate option?

G   The lateral lesion is one which, after wide local excision beyond the visible tumour edge, would not impinge upon the midline structures. Hence wide local excision with bilateral lymph node dissection is recommended.

A 56-year-old postmenopausal woman presents with a history of vulval itching and soreness of a few years' duration. On examination the vulva appears dry with scaly lesions throughout. Subsequent biopsy shows epithelial thinning and inflammatory changes suggesting lichen sclerosus. What is an appropriate option?

L   Potent steroids such as clobetasone are an effective treatment option for lichen sclerosus.

50 Management of adnexal mass

Answers: M F I C

An 18-year-old girl presents with urinary frequency. On examination she is found to have a lower abdominal mass. Ultrasound shows a 7 cm left-sided ovarian mass with mixed echogenicity. CT confirms the findings with fatty contents in the cyst, but no other pathology is seen. CA 125 and carcinoembryonic antigen levels are normal. What is an appropriate management option?

M   Mature teratomas are usually benign and common tumours in young girls. Definite treatment would depend upon the histopathology.

A 47-year-old perimenopausal lady had a pelvic scan for menorrhagia and was found to have a 4 cm anechoic thin-walled cyst. The CA 125 level is 18 units/mL. What is an appropriate management option?

F   A risk of malignancy index is used to assess the risk of benign ovarian cyst. Simple unilateral unilocular cyst can be managed by conservative methods.

A 54-year-old postmenopausal woman presents with an asymptomatic 4 cm ovarian cyst, which has persisted for a year. CA 125 level is normal. What is an appropriate management option?

I   If the cyst remains the same after a year (three scans), the patient can be discharged from follow-up.

A 32-year-old anxious lady presents with lower abdominal pain. She has a past history of irritable bowel syndrome. Pelvic ultrasound showed a 4 cm ovarian cyst, which was followed up 6 months later, when the cyst was reported to be 5 cm. Serum CA 125 was normal on both occasions. What is an appropriate management option?

C   Laparoscopic cystectomy can be performed in premenopausal women after discussion at a multidisciplinary team meeting.

51 Colposcopy

Answers: A D G D N

A 26-year-old lady is referred for colposcopy with mild dyskaryosis. Colposcopic examination suggests two areas of cervical intraepithelial neoplasia (CIN) I changes. What is appropriate management?

A   CIN I needs follow-up with repeat smear in 6 months.

A 50-year-old lady is referred with moderate dyskaryosis and is diagnosed with CIN II on colposcopy. What is appropriate management?

D   CIN II on colposcopy examination requires LLETZ. Further management would depend on the detailed histological examination of the specimen.

A 54-year-old Asian lady who has never had a smear presents with heavy bleeding and has a suspicious ulcerative lesion on her cervix. Further investigations reveal a stage III B cervical cancer.

G   Both chemoradiation and radiotherapy are treatment options for advanced cervical malignancy.

A 36-year-old lady is referred to colposcopy with severe dyskaryosis. On examination there are three acetowhite areas without uptake of iodine, suggestive of CIN III.

D   A LLETZ is therapeutic for CIN. Follow-up is required to check the completeness of excision.

A 45-year-old lady with known stage III cervical carcinoma presents with acute onset of heavy bleeding. She has bled through the vaginal pack. She is haemodynamically stable after an estimated 700 mL blood loss.

N   Radiotherapy is a treatment option in this emergency situation after initial resuscitation.

Section 8: Surgical gynaecology

52 Postoperative period investigations

53 Management of postoperative complications

54 Urinary tract injuries

55 Late postoperative complications

QUESTIONS

52 Postoperative period investigations

A flexible sigmoidoscopy
B barium enema
C computed tomography (CT) of the abdomen with rectal contrast
D midstream urine
E erect X-ray of the abdomen
F intravenous urogram
G cystoscopy
H blood cultures
I ventilation and perfusion scan
J chest X-ray
K electrocardiogram (ECG)
L take wound swabs and await the results
M serum urea and electrolytes
N examination under anaesthesia
O blood tests and troponin

For each description below, choose the **single** most appropriate answer from the above list of options. Each option may be used once, more than once, or not at all.

1 A 36-year-old lady had a laparoscopy for a persistent left-sided ovarian cyst. This was later converted to an open procedure. On the fourth postoperative day she complains of left-sided chest pain and fever. On chest examination she has bilateral equal air entry, with no added sounds. Abdominal examination is normal, and oxygen saturation is normal. What is the most appropriate investigation?

2 A 66-year-old lady had a vaginal hysterectomy for third-degree prolapse. On the first postoperative day she complains of left-sided chest pain and fever. She is tachycardic with a blood pressure of 100/70 mmHg. Clinical examination of the chest and abdomen are normal. Her haemoglobin is noted to be 11 g/dL. What is the most appropriate investigation?

3 A 36-year-old lady had a hysterectomy for menorrhagia with an uneventful postoperative period, and was discharged on the fifth postoperative day. A week later she is readmitted with hematuria and left-sided loin pain. A midstream urine sample arranged by her GP is negative. What is the most appropriate investigation?

4 A 40-year-old lady had a total abdominal hysterectomy for a benign ovarian cyst. On the third postoperative day she feels unwell with profuse vomiting, abdominal distension and no audible bowel sounds. C-Reactive protein (CRP), white cell count and haemoglobin levels are all normal. What is the most appropriate investigation?

5 A 58-year-old woman who is a chronic smoker underwent a total abdominal hysterectomy with bilateral salpingo-oophorectomy for persistent ovarian cyst.

Intraoperatively she developed myocardial infarction and needed to be intubated. She was in the intensive care unit and later transferred to the high-dependency unit postoperatively. On the 10th postoperative day she was noted to have a serous discharge from the wound with a 0.5 cm opening in the wound. She has been on antibiotics for a week. She is afebrile and the initial blood results (white cell count and CRP) are normal. What is the most appropriate investigation?

Answers: see page 110.

53 Management of postoperative complications

A   intravenous antibiotics
B   re-exploration of the abdomen
C   nephrostomy with or without stenting
D   blood transfusion
E   ultrasound-guided aspiration
F   chest physiotherapy
G   10 000 IU heparin followed by 5000 IU heparin subcutaneously
H   supportive measures
I   triple swab test
J   wound exploration and resuturing of the wound
K   streptokinase
L   nasogastric tube, intravenous fluids and correction of electrolytes
M   embolectomy

For each description below, choose the **single** most appropriate answer from the above list of options. Each option may be used once, more than once, or not at all.

1   A 38-year-old lady had a difficult abdominal hysterectomy for severe endometriosis. On the third postoperative day she felt unwell and developed a spiking fever of over 38.2°C on two occasions. She is on intravenous cefuroxime and metronidazole. On examination she is dehydrated, peripherally shut down and shocked. There is generalised abdominal tenderness with guarding and rigidity. A computed tomography scan with rectal contrast showed multiple fluid levels.

2   A 36-year-old lady had a laparoscopy for a persistent left-sided ovarian cyst. This was later converted to an open procedure. On the third postoperative day she complained of left-sided chest pain and fever. Chest examination and abdominal examination are normal. The chest X-ray shows patchy haziness over the right lower lobe. Oxygen saturation is 98 per cent. Her electrocardiogram is normal.

3   A 40-year-old lady had a total abdominal hysterectomy for a benign serous cystadenoma. On the third postoperative day she felt unwell with profuse vomiting. On examination there is tense abdominal distension. Initial blood test results are normal. An abdominal X-ray shows multiple fluid levels.

4   A 58-year-old chronic smoker underwent a total abdominal hysterectomy with bilateral salpingo-oophorectomy for a persistent ovarian cyst. Intraoperatively she developed a myocardial infarction and needed to be ventilated. She was in the intensive care unit and was later transferred to the high-dependency unit postoperatively. On the 10th postoperative day she was noted to have a serous discharge from the wound, which was sent for culture. She has been on antibiotics for a week. She is afebrile and the initial blood results were normal. After 2 days she is noted to have complete wound dehiscence.

Answers: see page 111.

54 Urinary tract injuries

A suprapubic catheter
B uretero-neocystostomy
C renal ultrasound
D intraoperative cystoscopy
E suprapubic catheter and Foley catheter
F double-layered closure and continuous bladder drainage for 1 week
G end-to-end anastomosis with a stent
H end-to-end anastomosis
I Boari flab
J CT urogram
K intraoperative cystoscopy
L expectant management
M uretero-ureterostomy
N cystoscopy
O percutaneous nephrostomy

For each description below, choose the **single** most appropriate answer from the above list of options. Each option may be used once, more than once, or not at all.

1 A 52-year-old lady undergoes a laparotomy for suspected ovarian malignancy. Her left ureter is inadvertently injured during ligation of the infundibulopelvic ligament. A complete transection of the mid-ureter is noted. What is the appropriate surgical management?

2 A 27-year-old lady undergoes a repeat elective caesarean section under general anaesthetic for previous two lower-segment caesarean sections. At the end of the surgery urine is noted to be heavily bloodstained and a 2 cm rent in the bladder is noted. What is the appropriate surgical management?

3 A 37-year-old lady undergoes a hysterectomy for multiple fibroids. The anatomy of the pelvis is distorted and the right ureter is inadvertently clamped while a blind bleeding spot is noted near the uterine vessels. It is immediately recognised and the clamp released. What is the appropriate surgical management?

4 A 34-year-old woman undergoes a laparotomy for severe bilateral endometriosis. During the operation, the right ureter is involved in a needle injury. No obvious damage to the ureter is noted. What is the next step?

Answers: see page 111.

55 Late postoperative complications

A   pelvic floor exercises
B   tension-free tape
C   ultrasound-guided aspiration
D   counselling
E   observation
F   analgesics, antibiotics and follow-up
G   midstream urine culture
H   computed tomography urogram/intravenous pyelogram
I   repair of an incisional hernia
J   re-laparotomy
K   antibiotics and repeat ultrasound
L   hormone replacement therapy (HRT)
M   repair with Prolene mesh
N   expectant management

For each description below, choose the **single** most appropriate answer from the above list of options. Each option may be used once, more than once, or not at all.

1   A 48-year-old lady underwent tension-free vaginal tape (TVT) management for stress incontinence. She attends the 6-week follow-up clinic and is still complaining of leakage while sneezing and coughing.

2   A 54-year-old nulliparous woman underwent vaginal hysterectomy and pelvic floor repair. Postoperatively she was treated for a *Klebsiella* urine infection. Five weeks after her operation she complains of diarrhoea and tenesmus. On examination the vault appears healthy. There is an 8 × 8 cm-size fluid collection in the pelvis. What is appropriate management?

3   A 37-year-old lady underwent total abdominal hysterectomy with ovarian conservation for multiple fibroids. She was discharged on the fifth postoperative day. She has been treated for urinary tract infection (UTI) on two occasions by her GP. She attends the 6-week follow-up and complains of a persistent loss of watery fluid from her vagina.

4   A 46-year-old lady underwent total abdominal hysterectomy and bilateral salpingo-oophorectomy for severe endometriosis. She attends the 6-week postoperative follow-up and complains of severe hot flushes.

Answers: see page 112.

ANSWERS

52 Postoperative period investigations

Answers: J K F E L

A 36-year-old lady had a laparoscopy for a persistent left-sided ovarian cyst. This was later converted to an open procedure. On the fourth postoperative day she complains of left-sided chest pain and fever. On chest examination she has bilateral equal air entry, with no added sounds. Abdominal examination is normal, and oxygen saturation is normal. What is the most appropriate investigation?

J   Pneumonia, pulmonary atelectasis and pulmonary embolism are the differential diagnoses. A chest X-ray is the appropriate investigation of choice.

A 66-year-old lady had a vaginal hysterectomy for third-degree prolapse. On the first postoperative day she complains of left-sided chest pain and fever. She is tachycardic with a blood pressure of 100/70 mmHg. Clinical examination of the chest and abdomen are normal. Her haemoglobin is noted to be 11 g/dL. What is the most appropriate investigation?

K   Ischaemic heart disease needs to be ruled out in this scenario. ECG followed by blood tests for cardiac enzymes are the appropriate investigations. Although pulmonary embolism is possible, it is less likely in the early postoperative period.

A 36-year-old lady had a hysterectomy for menorrhagia with an uneventful postoperative period, and was discharged on the fifth postoperative day. A week later she is readmitted with hematuria and left-sided loin pain. A midstream urine sample arranged by her GP is negative. What is the most appropriate investigation?

F   Ureteric injuries occur in about 0.1–2.5 per cent. Both an intravenous urogram and a CT urogram could be considered in these situations.

A 40-year-old lady had a total abdominal hysterectomy for a benign ovarian cyst. On the third postoperative day she feels unwell with profuse vomiting, abdominal distension and no audible bowel sounds. C-Reactive protein (CRP), white cell count and haemoglobin levels are all normal. What is the most appropriate investigation?

E   Paralytic ileus is the likely diagnosis, and an abdominal X-ray is helpful.

A 58-year-old woman who is a chronic smoker underwent a total abdominal hysterectomy with bilateral salpingo-oophorectomy for persistent ovarian cyst. Intraoperatively she developed myocardial infarction and needed to be intubated. She was in the intensive care unit and later transferred to the high-dependency unit postoperatively. On the 10th postoperative day she was noted to have a serous discharge from the wound with a 0.5 cm opening in the wound. She has been on antibiotics for a week. She is afebrile and the initial blood results (white cell count and CRP) are normal. What is the most appropriate investigation?

L   Treating the underlying wound infection will suffice a small wound dehiscence.

53 Management of postoperative complications

Answers: B A L J

A 38-year-old lady had a difficult abdominal hysterectomy for severe endometriosis. On the third postoperative day she felt unwell and developed a spiking fever of over 38.2ºC on two occasions. She is on intravenous cefuroxime and metronidazole. On examination she is dehydrated, peripherally shut down and shocked. There is generalised abdominal tenderness with guarding and rigidity. A computed tomography scan with rectal contrast showed multiple fluid levels.

B   The incidence of bowel damage is quoted to be between 0.3 and 0.8 per cent after gynaecological surgery. Septic peritonitis is the likely diagnosis, and re-laparotomy and appropriate bowel repair by a suitably experienced surgeon are indicated.

A 36-year-old lady had a laparoscopy for a persistent left-sided ovarian cyst. This was later converted to an open procedure. On the third postoperative day she complained of left-sided chest pain and fever. Chest examination and abdominal examination are normal. The chest X-ray shows patchy haziness over the right lower lobe. Oxygen saturation is 98 per cent. Her electrocardiogram is normal.

A   Pneumonia could complicate the postoperative period and needs aggressive treatment with antibiotics and chest physiotherapy.

A 40-year-old lady had a total abdominal hysterectomy for a benign serous cystadenoma. On the third postoperative day she felt unwell with profuse vomiting. On examination there is tense abdominal distension. Initial blood test results are normal. An abdominal X-ray shows multiple fluid levels.

L   A paralytic ileus usually improves with nasogastric tube aspiration, intravenous fluids and correction of electrolytes.

A 58-year-old chronic smoker underwent a total abdominal hysterectomy with bilateral salpingo-oophorectomy for a persistent ovarian cyst. Intraoperatively she developed a myocardial infarction and needed to be ventilated. She was in the intensive care unit and was later transferred to the high-dependency unit postoperatively. On the 10th postoperative day she was noted to have a serous discharge from the wound, which was sent for culture. She has been on antibiotics for a week. She is afebrile and the initial blood results were normal. After 2 days she is noted to have complete wound dehiscence.

J   A large wound dehiscence needs surgical exploration and repair.

54 Urinary tract injuries

Answers: G F D L

A 52-year-old lady undergoes a laparotomy for suspected ovarian malignancy. Her left ureter is inadvertently injured during ligation of the infundibulopelvic ligament. A complete transection of the mid-ureter is noted. What is the appropriate surgical management?

G   Intraoperative ureteric injuries are best managed by immediate repair.

A 27-year-old lady undergoes a repeat elective caesarean section under general anaesthetic for previous two lower-segment caesarean sections. At the end of the surgery urine is noted to be heavily bloodstained and a 2 cm rent in the bladder is noted. What is the appropriate surgical management?

F   Uncomplicated bladder injury carries a better prognosis if it is recognised and repaired in two layers.

A 37-year-old lady undergoes a hysterectomy for multiple fibroids. The anatomy of the pelvis is distorted and the right ureter is inadvertently clamped while a blind bleeding spot is noted near the uterine vessels. It is immediately recognised and the clamp released. What is the appropriate surgical management?

D   Intravenous administration of dye (indigo carmine) followed by cystoscopy is useful in assessing the ureteric damage.

A 34-year-old woman undergoes a laparotomy for severe bilateral endometriosis. During the operation, the right ureter is involved in a needle injury. No obvious damage to the ureter is noted. What is the next step?

L   Uncomplicated needle injury to the ureter without obvious bleeding or leaking needs no active surgical management.

55 Late postoperative complications

Answers: A C H L

A 48-year-old lady underwent tension-free vaginal tape (TVT) management for stress incontinence. She attends the 6-week follow-up clinic and is still complaining of leakage while sneezing and coughing.

A   The success rate of TVT as an initial procedure is reported to be about 85–90 per cent. Pelvic floor exercises should be offered initially at this stage.

A 54-year-old nulliparous woman underwent vaginal hysterectomy and pelvic floor repair. Postoperatively she was treated for a *Klebsiella* urine infection. Five weeks after her operation she complains of diarrhoea and tenesmus. On examination the vault appears healthy. There is an 8 × 8 cm-size fluid collection in the pelvis. What is appropriate management?

C   A symptomatic pelvic collection could be drained either by ultrasound guidance or in theatre.

A 37-year-old lady underwent total abdominal hysterectomy with ovarian conservation for multiple fibroids. She was discharged on the fifth postoperative day. She has been treated for urinary tract infection (UTI) on two occasions by her GP. She attends the 6-week follow-up and complains of a persistent loss of watery fluid from her vagina.

H   Recurrent UTIs and persistent watery loss can be sign of an underlying fistula and needs further investigation.

A 46-year-old lady underwent total abdominal hysterectomy and bilateral salpingo-oophorectomy for severe endometriosis. She attends the 6-week postoperative follow-up and complains of severe hot flushes.

L   Detailed counselling regarding HRT and subsequent reactivation of endometriosis is necessary.

Section 9: Subfertility

56 Management of subfertility

57 Causes of subfertility

58 Investigation of amenorrhoea

QUESTIONS

56 Management of subfertility

A laparoscopic ovarian drilling

B metroplasty

C surrogacy

D adoption

E ovum donation

F intracytoplasmic sperm injection (ICSI)/in vitro fertilisation (IVF)

G in vitro fertilisation

H tubal reconstructive surgery

I clomiphene

J metformin

K weight reduction

L laparoscopic ablation of endometriosis/ovarian cystectomy

M intrauterine insemination

N donor insemination

O gamete intrafallopian tube transfer

For each description below, choose the **single** most appropriate answer from the above list of options. Each option may be used once, more than once, or not at all.

1 A couple are seen in infertility clinic for follow-up of their results. The female partner has a normal day 21 progesterone level. Hysterosalpingography (HSG) shows bilateral patent tubes. Repeat semen analysis shows a volume of 2.8 ml, a pH of 7.4 and a sperm count of 3×10^6 million/ml. The couple are very keen on being genetic parents.

2 A 34-year-old woman with a body mass index (BMI) of 26 has a day 23 progesterone level of 10 nmol/L. HSG shows bilateral patent tubes. Her partner's semen analysis shows a volume of 3 ml, a pH of 7 and a sperm count of 20×10^6 million/ml. She had tried 6 months of clomiphene with documented anovulation. A trial of metformin was not successful. What is the next appropriate step?

3 A 31-year-old lady is seen in the subfertility clinic. She has a long history of deep dyspareunia. Her partner's semen analysis shows a volume of 3 mL, a pH of 7 and a sperm count of 20×10^6 million/ml. Ovulation is confirmed with day 21 progesterone. Previous laparoscopy showed stage 2 endometriosis. What is the next appropriate step?

4 A 34-year-old lady presents with a 2-year history of amenorrhoea. Her partner's semen analysis is normal. Tubal patency is confirmed on HSG. Her serum

luteinising hormone level is 100 units/L and her follicle-stimulating hormone level is 120 units/L. She is medically fit and healthy. What is the next appropriate step?

5   A 24-year-old woman presents with a 3-year history of subfertility. Investigations show bilateral patent tubes, there is a day 21 progesterone of 18 nmol/L and her partner's semen analysis is reported as normal. Her BMI is 37. What is the next appropriate step?

Answers: see page 120.

57 Causes of subfertility

A endometriosis
B oligospermia
C Kallman's syndrome
D premature ovarian failure
E anovulatory subfertility
F polycystic ovarian syndrome
G prolactinoma
H cervical factor infertility
I Asherman's syndrome
J oligoasthenospermia
K Young's syndrome
L müllerian agenesis
M coital dysfunction
N azoospermia
O tubal factor infertility

For each description below, choose the **single** most appropriate answer from the above list of options. Each option may be used once, more than once, or not at all.

1 A couple present with a 2-year history of subfertility. The results of the female partner include a luteinising hormone (LH) of 4.6 units/L, a follicle-stimulating hormone (FSH) of 3.2 units/L and a prolactin of 440 units/L. The day 21 progesterone is 12 nmol/L. Hysterosalpingography (HSG) shows patent tubes. Semen analysis shows a count of 40×10^6 million/ml with normal forms greater than 50 per cent, 50 per cent forward progression, and no evidence of agglutination or white blood cells.

2 A couple present to the subfertility clinic for results. The female partner has an FSH of 6.1 IU/L, an LH of 4.8 IU/L, a prolactin of 210 nmol/L and a day 21 progesterone of 38 nmol/L. Laparoscopy 6 months ago showed a normal pelvis. She is awaiting HSG. Semen analysis results were as follows: volume 3 mL, sperm count 10×10^6 million/ml, 18 per cent forward progression with motility and normal forms greater than 50 per cent. No agglutination or white cells were found. No organisms were seen.

3 A 29-year-old woman presents with secondary subfertility. She had a spontaneous miscarriage 3 years ago followed by an ectopic pregnancy. She was treated for chlamydial infection 4 years ago. She suffers from deep dyspareunia. Her partner's semen analysis results have been normal on two occasions. Her day 21 progesterone level is 35 nmol/L, her FSH 4.6 IU/L and her LH 3.1 IU/L.

4 A 25-year-old woman presents to the subfertility clinic with irregular periods and recent amenorrhoea of 6 months. Her partner's semen analysis has been reported to be normal. She also suffers from excessive acne and hair loss. Tubal patency is normal on HSG. What is the most likely cause?

5   A 31-year-old lady presents with secondary subfertility. She had difficulty con-
    ceiving her first child and has now been trying for 4 years. She gives a history of
    cyclical premenstrual pain, painful periods and deep dyspareunia. Her day 21
    progesterone is 38 nmol/L with normal levels of FSH and LH. What is the most
    likely cause?

Answers: see page 120.

58 Investigation of amenorrhoea

A glucose tolerance test
B luteinising hormone (LH)/follicle-stimulating hormone (FSH) and free androgen index
C buccal smear/karyotyping
D pregnancy test
E serum prolactin
F serum progesterone
G serum oestradiol
H testosterone and sex hormone-binding globulin (SHBG)
I Synacthen test
J serum adrenocorticotrophic hormone (ACTH)
K serum cortisol
L serum insulin
M thyroid-stimulating hormone (TSH)/thyroxine
N visual field examination
O computed tomography of the head

For each description below, choose the **single** most appropriate answer from the above list of options. Each option may be used once, more than once, or not at all.

1   A 44-year-old lady presents with 4 months' amenorrhoea. She also complains of easy fatigability. She gives a history of 6 months' amenorrhoea 15 months ago when she was investigated and discharged with normal results. Her GP had organised blood tests, which showed normal LH and FSH, raised prolactin, normal testosterone and SHBG. She had a borderline raised TSH and thyroxine. What is the next appropriate investigation?

2   A 25-year-old lady presents with a 6-month history of secondary amenorrhoea. Her height is 10 cm below her mid-parental height. She has a negative pregnancy test. She started menarche at 18 years of age. She is noted to have a short neck and a wide carrying angle. What is the most relevant investigation to establish the diagnosis?

3   A 23-year-old lady presents with 8 months' amenorrhoea and excessive hair loss with an appearance of facial hair. Two months previously there had been bereavement in the family. She has a negative pregnancy test. What is the most appropriate investigation?

4   A 19-year-old girl presents with a recent onset of facial hair growth and 4 months' history of secondary amenorrhoea. Investigations by her GP showed a negative pregnancy test and normal LH, FSH and thyroid function test results. Pelvic ultrasound and blood glucose were normal. Serum androgen was elevated. What would be the next appropriate test?

Answers: see page 121.

ANSWERS

56 Management of subfertility

Answers: F A L E K

A couple are seen in infertility clinic for follow-up of their results. The female partner has a normal day 21 progesterone level. Hysterosalpingography (HSG) shows bilateral patent tubes. Repeat semen analysis shows a volume of 2.8 ml, a pH of 7.4 and a sperm count of 3×10^6 million/ml. The couple are very keen on being genetic parents.

F Severe oligospermia and azoospermia will be an indication for ICSI/IVF.

A 34-year-old woman with a body mass index (BMI) of 26 has a day 23 progesterone level of 10 nmol/L. HSG shows bilateral patent tubes. Her partner's semen analysis shows a volume of 3 ml, a pH of 7 and a sperm count of 20×10^6 million/ml. She had tried 6 months of clomiphene with documented anovulation. A trial of metformin was not successful. What is the next appropriate step?

A Ovarian drilling may be offered for clomiphene-resistant cases.

A 31-year-old lady is seen in the subfertility clinic. She has a long history of deep dyspareunia. Her partner's semen analysis shows a volume of 3 mL, a pH of 7 and a sperm count of 20×10^6 million/ml. Ovulation is confirmed with day 21 progesterone. Previous laparoscopy showed stage 2 endometriosis. What is the next appropriate step?

L Treatment of stage 1–2 endometriosis associated with subfertility by resection or ablation has been shown to improve outcome.

A 34-year-old lady presents with a 2-year history of amenorrhoea. Her partner's semen analysis is normal. Tubal patency is confirmed on HSG. Her serum luteinising hormone level is 100 units/L and her follicle-stimulating hormone level is 120 units/L. She is medically fit and healthy. What is the next appropriate step?

E In premature menopause ovum donation is an option. Surrogacy and adoption could also be considered.

A 24-year-old woman presents with a 3-year history of subfertility. Investigations show bilateral patent tubes, there is a day 21 progesterone of 18 nmol/L and her partner's semen analysis is reported as normal. Her BMI is 37. What is the next appropriate step?

K If the BMI is greater than 30 and the patient has oligomenorrhoea, weight reduction is initially advised before medical treatment.

57 Causes of subfertility

Answers: E J O F A

A couple present with a 2-year history of subfertility. The results of the female partner include a luteinising hormone (LH) of 4.6 IU/L, a follicle-stimulating hormone (FSH) of 3.2 IU/L and a prolactin of 440 units/L. The day 21 progesterone is

12 nmol/L. Hysterosalpingography (HSG) shows patent tubes. Semen analysis shows a count of 40×10^6 million/ml with normal forms greater than 50 per cent, 50 per cent forward progression, and no evidence of agglutination or white blood cells.

E   A day 21 progesterone of greater than 30 nmol/L is considered to be indicative of ovulation.

A couple present to the subfertility clinic for results. The female partner has an FSH of 6.1 IU/L, an LH of 4.8 IU/L, a prolactin of 210 nmol/L and a day 21 progesterone of 38 nmol/L. Laparoscopy 6 months ago showed a normal pelvis. She is awaiting HSG. Semen analysis results were as follows: volume 3 mL, sperm count 10×10^6 million/ml, 18 per cent forward progression with motility and normal forms greater than 50 per cent. No agglutination or white cells were found. No organisms were seen.

J   Sperm counts of 20 million/mL or more, with 50 per cent or more motile and 25 per cent or more with forward motility are considered to be normal results.

A 29-year-old woman presents with secondary subfertility. She had a spontaneous miscarriage 3 years ago followed by an ectopic pregnancy. She was treated for chlamydial infection 4 years ago. She suffers from deep dyspareunia. Her partner's semen analysis results have been normal on two occasions. Her day 21 progesterone level is 35 nmol/L, her FSH 4.6 IU/L and her LH 3.1 IU/L.

O   Previous ectopic pregnancy and chlamydial infection would suggest tubal factors as the cause of her infertility.

A 25-year-old woman presents to the subfertility clinic with irregular periods and recent amenorrhoea of 6 months. Her partner's semen analysis has been reported to be normal. She also suffers from excessive acne and hair loss. Tubal patency is normal on HSG. What is the most likely cause?

F   Polycystic ovarian syndrome can be diagnosed if two of the following three factors are present: evidence of hyperandrogenism, ovulatory dysfunction or morphological polycystic ovaries.

A 31-year-old lady presents with secondary subfertility. She had difficulty conceiving her first child and has now been trying for 4 years. She gives a history of cyclical premenstrual pain, painful periods and deep dyspareunia. Her day 21 progesterone is 38 nmol/L with normal levels of FSH and LH. What is the most likely cause?

A   Dysmenorrhoea, deep dyspareunia and secondary subfertility suggest endometriosis as the underlying cause.

58 Investigation of amenorrhoea

Answers: D C H I

A 44-year-old lady presents with 4 months' amenorrhoea. She also complains of easy fatigability. She gives a history of 6 months' amenorrhoea 15 months ago when she was investigated and discharged with normal results. Her GP had organised blood tests, which showed normal LH and FSH, raised prolactin, normal testosterone and SHBG. She had a borderline raised TSH and thyroxine. What is the next appropriate investigation?

D   Any history of amenorrhoea in the reproductive age group must initiate a pregnancy test.

A 25-year-old lady presents with a 6-month history of secondary amenorrhoea. Her height is 10 cm below her mid-parental height. She has a negative pregnancy test. She started menarche at 18 years of age. She is noted to have a short neck and a wide carrying angle. What is the most relevant investigation to establish the diagnosis?

C   Short stature with amenorrhoea should prompt a diagnosis of Turner's syndrome. It can occasionally present with secondary amenorrhoea.

A 23-year-old lady presents with 8 months' amenorrhoea and excessive hair loss with an appearance of facial hair. Two months previously there had been bereavement in the family. She has a negative pregnancy test. What is the most appropriate investigation?

H   Stress-related hair loss occurs after 6 months. Amenorrhoea and alopecia may be a presentation of polycystic ovarian syndrome.

A 19-year-old girl presents with a recent onset of facial hair growth and 4 months' history of secondary amenorrhoea. Investigations by her GP showed a negative pregnancy test and normal LH, FSH and thyroid function test results. Pelvic ultrasound and blood glucose were normal. Serum androgen was elevated. What would be the next appropriate test?

I   Late-onset congenital adrenal hyperplasia is a known cause of hirsutism. Normal tests for polycystic ovarian syndrome other than androgens should prompt a Synacthen test.

Section 10: Urogynaecology

59 Diagnosis of urinary conditions

60 Management options in urogynaecology

QUESTIONS

59 Diagnosis of urinary conditions

A   stress incontinence
B   overactive bladder
C   drug-induced diuresis
D   urodynamic stress incontinence
E   outflow tract obstruction
F   urinary tract infection
G   sensory bladder
H   mass compressing the bladder
I   uterine incarceration
J   vesicovaginal fistula
K   neuropathic bladder
L   nocturnal enuresis
M   colovesical fistula
N   interstitial cystitis
O   spinal cord compression

For each description below, choose the **single** most appropriate answer from the above list of options. Each option may be used once, more than once, or not at all.

1   A 36-year-old Afro-Caribbean lady presents with a pregnancy at 12 weeks' gestation with severe abdominal pain and not having voided for the past 10 hours. On examination the uterus is retroverted. What is the most likely diagnosis?

2   A 64-year-old Asian lady presents with heavy postmenopausal bleeding. She has never had a smear. An ulcerative lesion is found on her cervix. She complains of leaking clear fluid through the vagina. What is the most likely diagnosis?

3   A 45-year-old lady who is para 3 and is a gym instructor presents with complaints of leakage of urine during exercise. A subsequent urodynamic study shows a normal bladder capacity, a free flow of 18 mL per second and a stable bladder. What is the most likely diagnosis?

4   A 66-year-old lady presents with a history of difficulty in micturition. She voids three times a day with large volumes. She has no stress symptoms or urgency. Urodynamic study shows a flow rate of 3 mL per second, a bladder capacity of 800 mL and a voiding time of 320 seconds. Her first desire to void is at 400 mL, her second desire to void at 600 mL and urgency at 800 mL. What is the most likely diagnosis?

Answers: see page 126.

60 Management options in urogynaecology

A anterior colporrhaphy
B vaginal hysterectomy and pelvic floor repair
C Burch colposuspension
D tension-free vaginal tape
E collagen injection
F ambulatory urodynamics
G pelvic floor exercises
H weight reduction
I diabetes screening
J artificial sphincter
K tolterodine
L duloxetine
M oxybutynin
N a device to block the external meatus
O topical oestrogens
P do nothing

For each description below, choose the **single** most appropriate answer from the above list of options. Each option may be used once, more than once, or not at all.

1 A 23-year-old lady who is para 2 presents with a 6-month history of stress incontinence. Her body mass index is 34. She had a caesarean section 11 months ago for breech presentation. What is the most appropriate management?

2 A 40-year-old lady who is para 2 is diagnosed with urodynamic stress incontinence. She has tried pelvic floor exercises but has not found it to be useful. She is a fitness instructor. What is the most appropriate management?

3 A 42-year-old para 2 lady presents for her smear and is found to have an asymptomatic cystocele. What is the most appropriate management?

Answers: see page 126.

ANSWERS

59 Diagnosis of urinary conditions

Answers: I J D E

A 36-year-old Afro-Caribbean lady presents with a pregnancy at 12 weeks' gestation with severe abdominal pain and not having voided for the past 10 hours. On examination the uterus is retroverted. What is the most likely diagnosis?

I   An acutely retroverted uterus can cause urinary retention at the beginning of the second trimester. Immediate relief occurs after catheterisation. The condition is self-limiting and improves with advancing gestation.

A 64-year-old Asian lady presents with heavy postmenopausal bleeding. She has never had a smear. An ulcerative lesion is found on her cervix. She complains of leaking clear fluid through the vagina. What is the most likely diagnosis?

J   Vesicovaginal fistula is a complication of advanced cervical malignancy.

A 45-year-old lady who is para 3 and is a gym instructor presents with complaints of leakage of urine during exercise. A subsequent urodynamic study shows a normal bladder capacity, a free flow of 18 mL per second and a stable bladder. What is the most likely diagnosis?

D   Urodynamic stress incontinence is defined as the presence of urinary incontinence associated with a rise in intra-abdominal pressure, in the absence of detrusor contraction.

A 66-year-old lady presents with a history of difficulty in micturition. She voids three times a day with large volumes. She has no stress symptoms or urgency. Urodynamic study shows a flow rate of 3 mL per second, a bladder capacity of 800 mL and a voiding time of 320 seconds. Her first desire to void is at 400 mL, her second desire to void at 600 mL and urgency at 800 mL. What is the most likely diagnosis?

E   Habitual chronic retention leads to a large capacity of the bladder. The normal flow rate is greater than 15 mL/second. Poor flow is suggestive of bladder outflow obstruction or poor detrusor function. Ureteric obstruction is associated with a high detrusor pressure on voiding, and poor detrusor function is associated with a low detrusor pressure.

60 Management options in urogynaecology

Answers: H D P

A 23-year-old lady who is para 2 presents with a 6-month history of stress incontinence. Her body mass index is 34. She had a caesarean section 11 months ago for breech presentation. What is the most appropriate management?

H   Weight reduction is the first line of treatment, with pelvic floor exercises.

A 40-year-old lady who is para 2 is diagnosed with urodynamic stress incontinence. She has tried pelvic floor exercises but has not found it to be useful. She is a fitness instructor. What is the most appropriate management?

D   Tension-free vaginal tape is the current gold standard for the treatment of urodynamic stress incontinence.

A 42-year-old para 2 lady presents for her smear and is found to have an asymptomatic cystocele. What is the most appropriate management?

P   Asymptomatic prolapse does not need treatment.

Section 11: Menopause and HRT

61 Postmenopausal bleeding

62 Choice of HRT

63 Choice of HRT

QUESTIONS

61 Postmenopausal bleeding

A total abdominal hysterectomy and bilateral salpingo-oophorectomy
B dilatation and curettage
C outpatient hysteroscopy and biopsy
D transcervical resection of the endometrium
E ultrasound pelvis
F Pipelle endometrial sampling
G a levonorgestrel-releasing intrauterine system
H rigid hysteroscopy and endometrial biopsy
I do nothing
J stop hormone replacement therapy (HRT)
K tibolone
L topical oestrogens
M change to raloxifene
N rigid hysteroscopy and polypectomy
O examination under anaesthesia

For each description below, choose the **single** most appropriate answer from the above list of options. Each option may be used once, more than once, or not at all.

1 A 64-year-old lady is on tamoxifen for her breast cancer. She is anxious about the information she has read in a women's magazine about the risk of endometrial cancer. She has no vaginal bleeding. What is the appropriate next step?

2 A 52-year-old parous lady has been on HRT for 3 years for vasomotor symptoms. Her periods have been irregular and erratic for the past 3 months. Ultrasound of the pelvis shows an endometrial thickness of 9 mm and normal adnexa. What is the appropriate next step?

3 A 72-year-old lady presents with postmenopausal bleeding/spotting lasting for the past 3 months. She also complains of vaginal bleeding and itching. She had a hysterectomy for a benign ovarian condition 20 years ago. Clinical examination is normal except for vaginal dryness. What is the appropriate next step?

4 A 48-year-old lady who is para 1 attends the gynaecology clinic for irregular and erratic bleeding occurring for the past 6 months. Ultrasound shows a normal uterus with an endometrial thickness of 4 mm. Her level of luteinising hormone is 4 units/L and her follicle-stimulating hormone is 6 units/L. What is the appropriate next step?

5 A 53-year-old lady who is para 3 presents with postmenopausal bleeding. Pelvic ultrasound shows an endometrial thickness of 16 mm with a rim of surrounding fluid. What is the appropriate next step?

6 An 84-year-old lady who lives in a care home has been noted to have blood in her underpants over the past month. She is also incontinent of urine. She is otherwise medically well. What is the appropriate next step?

Answers: see page 133.

62 Choice of HRT

A tibolone
B conjugated equine oestradiol
C raloxifene
D local oestrogens
E St John's wort
F progesterone for 14 days
G stop hormones
H a levonorgestrel-releasing intrauterine system
I dermovate cream
J exercises and stopping smoking
K cyclical oestrogens and progestogen
L biphosphonates
M lubricants
N clonidine
O 'bleed-free' combined oestrogen and progestogen therapy

For each description below, choose the **single** most appropriate answer from the above list of options. Each option may be used once, more than once, or not at all.

1 A 36-year-old lady undergoes total abdominal hysterectomy and bilateral salpingo-oophorectomy for painful complex adnexal masses. She is being seen in the gynaecology clinic 6 weeks later. The histology is reported to be benign. She is complaining of severe hot flushes. What is the most appropriate choice?

2 A 50-year-old executive complains of severe vasomotor symptoms, a lack of concentration and irritability. Her periods are regular and she was evaluated for perimenopausal bleeding 6 months ago. The results were found to be completely normal. What is the most appropriate choice?

3 A 55-year-old lady is complaining of dyspareunia and severe nocturia. A mid-stream urine culture is negative on two occasions. On examination the vulva and vagina appear dry. Vulval biopsies have shown no abnormalities. What is the most appropriate choice?

4 A 70-year-old lady is complaining of vulval soreness. On examination the vulva and vagina appear dry and thinned out. Histology shows hyperkeratosis in the stratum corneum and fibrosis in the dermis. She is medically fit otherwise. What is the most appropriate choice?

Answers: see page 134.

63 Choice of HRT

A tibolone
B conjugated equine oestradiol
C raloxifene
D local oestrogens
E St John's wort
F progesterone for 14 days
G stop hormones
H levonorgestrel-releasing intrauterine system
I dermovate cream
J exercise and stopping smoking
K cyclical oestrogens and progestogen
L biphosphonates
M lubricants
N clonidine
O 'bleed-free' combined oestrogen and progestogen therapy

For each description below, choose the **single** most appropriate answer from the above list of options. Each option may be used once, more than once, or not at all.

1 A 38-year-old lady underwent total abdominal hysterectomy and salpingo-oophorectomy for severe endometriosis. She now has severe vasomotor symptoms and requests advice on hormone replacement therapy (HRT).

2 A 56-year-old postmenopausal woman who is a chronic smoker attends the clinic for advice. She is worried about osteoporosis and requests HRT. What is the most appropriate advice?

3 A 40-year-old woman with oestrogen-receptor positive breast cancer treated with wide local excision followed by radiotherapy attends gynaecology clinic for advice regarding HRT. She is suffering from severe vasomotor symptoms.

4 A 51-year-old lady complains of severe hot flushes and sleeplessness. She had an inferior wall ischaemia the previous year and is on nitrates. She seeks advice regarding HRT. What is the most appropriate choice?

Answers: see page 134.

ANSWERS

61 Postmenopausal bleeding

Answers: I C L C N O

A 64-year-old lady is on tamoxifen for her breast cancer. She is anxious about the information she has read in a women's magazine about the risk of endometrial cancer. She has no vaginal bleeding. What is the appropriate next step?
I   No investigations are needed for women on tamoxifen with no bleeding.

A 52-year-old parous lady has been on HRT for 3 years for vasomotor symptoms. Her periods have been irregular and erratic for the past 3 months. Ultrasound of the pelvis shows an endometrial thickness of 9 mm and normal adnexa. What is the appropriate next step?
C   Women on HRT with an endometrial thickness more than 5 mm need further evaluation of endometrial histology.

A 72-year-old lady presents with postmenopausal bleeding/spotting lasting for the past 3 months. She also complains of vaginal bleeding and itching. She had a hysterectomy for a benign ovarian condition 20 years ago. Clinical examination is normal except for vaginal dryness. What is the appropriate next step?
L   Atrophic vaginitis, the most common cause of postmenopausal bleeding, is treated with local oestrogens without investigation in the absence of a uterus.

A 48-year-old lady who is para 1 attends the gynaecology clinic for irregular and erratic bleeding occurring for the past 6 months. Ultrasound shows a normal uterus with an endometrial thickness of 4 mm. Her level of luteinising hormone is 4 units/L and her follicle-stimulating hormone is 6 units/L. What is the appropriate next step?
C   Perimenopausal bleeding should be evaluated with endometrial histology. Endometrial thickness is not of much value in premenopausal women.

A 53-year-old lady who is para 3 presents with postmenopausal bleeding. Pelvic ultrasound shows an endometrial thickness of 16 mm with a rim of surrounding fluid. What is the appropriate next step?
N   Polyps need removal under effective anaesthesia. Increased endometrial thickness and fluid in a cavity suggest a polyp.

An 84-year-old lady who lives in a care home has been noted to have blood in her underpants over the past month. She is also incontinent of urine. She is otherwise medically well. What is the appropriate next step?
O   Bleeding of unknown origin needs examination under anaesthesia, cystoscopy, hysteroscopy and sigmoidoscopy.

62 Choice of HRT

Answers: B K D I

A 36-year-old lady undergoes total abdominal hysterectomy and bilateral salpingo-oophorectomy for painful complex adnexal masses. She is being seen in the gynaecology clinic 6 weeks later. The histology is reported to be benign. She is complaining of severe hot flushes. What is the most appropriate choice?

B   Oestrogens are indicated until the expectant age of menopause in women undergoing bilateral salpingo-oophorectomy.

A 50-year-old executive complains of severe vasomotor symptoms, a lack of concentration and irritability. Her periods are regular and she was evaluated for perimenopausal bleeding 6 months ago. The results were found to be completely normal. What is the most appropriate choice?

K   If a woman has not gone through the menopause but still complains of vasomotor symptoms, cyclical HRT is indicated.

A 55-year-old lady is complaining of dyspareunia and severe nocturia. A midstream urine culture is negative on two occasions. On examination the vulva and vagina appear dry. Vulval biopsies have shown no abnormalities. What is the most appropriate choice?

D   Atrophic vaginitis can be safely treated with local oestrogens.

A 70-year-old lady is complaining of vulval soreness. On examination the vulva and vagina appear dry and thinned out. Histology shows hyperkeratosis in the stratum corneum and fibrosis in the dermis. She is medically fit otherwise. What is the most appropriate choice?

I   Lichen sclerosus is a relatively common condition in postmenopausal women and can be treated with topical steroids.

63 Choice of HRT

Answers: B J N N

A 38-year-old lady underwent total abdominal hysterectomy and salpingo-oophorectomy for severe endometriosis. She now has severe vasomotor symptoms and requests advice on hormone replacement therapy (HRT).

B   HRT can be used in younger women who have experienced a premature menopause (younger than 40 years), unless contraindicated, for treating menopausal symptoms and preventing osteoporosis until the age of normal menopause.

A 56-year-old postmenopausal woman who is a chronic smoker attends the clinic for advice. She is worried about osteoporosis and requests HRT. What is the most appropriate advice?

J   HRT is no longer recommended as a first line of treatment for the universal prevention of osteoporosis. Diet and lifestyle changes are helpful. If there is a family or personal history of osteoporosis, measures such as biphosphonates or HRT may be considered. A dual-energy X-ray absorptiometry bone scan can be arranged to assess for osteopenia.

A 40-year-old woman with oestrogen-receptor positive breast cancer treated with wide local excision followed by radiotherapy attends gynaecology clinic for advice regarding HRT. She is suffering from severe vasomotor symptoms.

N   Oestrogen receptor-positive breast cancer is a definite contraindication to systemic HRT. Other measures, for example clonidine, may be tried.

A 51-year-old lady complains of severe hot flushes and sleeplessness. She had an inferior wall ischaemia the previous year and is on nitrates. She seeks advice regarding HRT. What is the most appropriate choice?

N   HRT is not recommended in the presence of ischaemic heart disease. Other measures such as clonidine may be helpful.

Section 12: Sexual health and contraception

64 Human immunodeficiency virus infection

65 Choice of contraception

66 Emergency contraception

67 Contraception

68 Termination of pregnancy

69 Sexually transmitted infections

HUMAN IMMUNODEFICIENCY VIRUS INFECTION

QUESTIONS

64 Human immunodeficiency virus infection

A   elective caesarean section
B   HAART
C   contact tracing
D   inform the GP and partner
E   barrier contraception
F   combined oral contraceptive pills
G   regular monitoring of CD4 cell count
H   sulphadiazine
I   HAART, elective caesarean section and avoiding breast-feeding
J   intrauterine devices
K   foscarnet
L   commence zidovudine
M   combined oral contraceptive pills and male condoms
N   intravenous trimethoprim and sulphamethoxazole
O   elective caesarean section and avoiding breast-feeding

For each description below, choose the **single** most appropriate answer from the above list of options. Each option may be used once, more than once, or not at all.

1   A 21-year-old university student attends the genitourinary medicine (GUM) clinic requesting a sexually transmitted infection screen as her previous boyfriend has recently been diagnosed with human immunodeficiency virus (HIV) infection. She is completely asymptomatic and otherwise fit and healthy. She is found to be HIV positive. Her CD4 count is 1000 cells/mm³. Swabs for other sexually transmitted infections are negative. She is counselled fully about the diagnosis. What is the most suitable next step in her management?

2   A 28-year-old woman attends the GUM clinic. She is a known HIV-positive patient. Her most recent blood tests have shown normal liver function tests and a CD4 cell count of 500 cells/mm³. She is currently on GUM follow-up. She states that she is 6 months pregnant and has not so far had any antenatal checks. What is the most appropriate treatment option?

3   A 36-year-old intravenous drug user attends the Accident and Emergency department with a dry cough and breathlessness. Her chest X-ray shows bilateral perihilar interstitial shadows. She was first diagnosed with HIV infection 2 years ago, and is being followed up with blood results. She has recently defaulted treatment. Her CD4 count is 100 cells/mm³. What is the best management option?

4   A 28-year-old woman is seen in the sexual health clinic for contraceptive advice. She was diagnosed with HIV infection 2 months ago. Her CD4 count is 800 cells/mm³. She is completely asymptomatic. What is the most appropriate method of contraception?

Answers: see page 144.

137

SEXUAL HEALTH AND CONTRACEPTION

65 Choice of contraception

A   depot provera
B   a levonorgestrel intrauterine system
C   double Dutch method
D   male condoms
E   Implanon
F   tubal clip application
G   combined oral contraception
H   minipill
I   copper intrauterine contraceptive device (IUCD)
J   emergency contraception with the pill
K   female condoms
L   combined contraceptive patch
M   vasectomy
N   natural methods
O   spermicidal foam

For each description below, choose the **single** most appropriate answer from the above list of options. Each option may be used once, more than once, or not at all.

1   An 18-year-old girl requests contraception. She has been sexually active for 2 years and has been in a new relationship for the past 3 weeks. What is the most appropriate option?

2   A 34-year-old lady requests contraception. Her body mass index (BMI) is 35. She suffers from painful heavy periods. She thinks she has completed her family. She smokes 10 cigarettes a day. What is the most appropriate option?

3   A 29-year-old lady with a BMI of 37 who is para 4 is requesting permanent contraception. She fell pregnant on the combined oral contraceptive pill, and her periods are normal and last for 5 days. She had an intrauterine contraceptive device in the past and did not like it. She is worried about weight gain with Implanon and depot progesterone. What is the most appropriate option?

4   A 42-year-old lady who is para 3 requests contraception. She has been on the combined oral contraceptive pill for many years. She has recently become forgetful and requests an alternate non-hormonal long-term method. What is the most appropriate option?

5   A 26-year-old lady gave birth to a baby a month ago and is breast-feeding the baby. She was on the combined pill before and had no complaints with that. She has needle phobia and requests a short-term contraceptive. What is the most appropriate option?

Answers: see page 144.

66 Emergency contraception

A levonorgestrel two tablets stat
B reassurance
C levonorgestrel one tablet followed by a second tablet 12 hours later
D copper intrauterine contraceptive device
E contact tracing
F levonorgestrel-releasing intrauterine system
G resume pills
H copper IUCD and a pregnancy test in 2 weeks' time
I levonorgestrel two tablets stat and a pregnancy test if there has been no period in 2 weeks' time
J azithromycin 1 g stat
K Yuzpe method
L levonorgestrel two tablets stat, offer a full sexually transmitted infection screen and a pregnancy test if there has been no period in 2 weeks' time
M triple swabs
N pregnancy test
O intravenous antibiotics

For each description below, choose the **single** most appropriate answer from the above list of options. Each option may be used once, more than once, or not at all.

1 A 20-year-old girl attends the family planning clinic 6 hours after unprotected sexual intercourse. Her periods are regular and the first day of her last menstrual period was 3 weeks ago. Her current contraceptive method is male condoms. She also recalls another episode of condom split 10 days ago. Her pregnancy test is negative. What is the most appropriate advice?

2 A 27-year-old lady attends the family planning clinic 7 days after unprotected sexual intercourse. Her menstrual cycles are very regular (3–4/28). Her last menstrual period was 2 weeks ago. What is the most appropriate option?

3 A 37-year-old woman attends the clinic 6 hours after unprotected sexual intercourse. She suffers from idiopathic thrombocytopenic purpura and is on long-term steroids. Her periods are regular but heavy, and the first day of her last menstrual period was 2 weeks ago. What is the most appropriate option?

4 A 23-year-old nulliparous woman attends Accident and Emergency. She gives a history of unprotected sexual intercourse the previous night. Her periods are regular (3–4/30). She had sexual intercourse with a stranger. Her last menstrual period was 2 weeks ago. What is the most appropriate step?

5 A 19-year-old girl requests emergency contraception. She gives a history of unprotected sexual intercourse 40 hours ago. She is unsure of when her last menstrual period was as her periods are irregular. Her regular contraceptive method is the male condom. What is the first step in management?

Answers: see page 145.

67 Contraception

A change Implanon
B weight reduction
C counselling and reassurance
D pregnancy test
E triple swabs
F contact tracing
G other LARC methods (long-acting reversible contraceptive methods)
H change the copper coil
I outpatient endometrial sampling
J remove the intrauterine contraceptive device (IUCD) and repeat triple swabs
K doxycycline 100 mg twice daily for 14 days
L remove Implanon and start combined pills
M remove the IUCD, hysteroscopy and curettage
N azithromycin 1 g stat
O stop the combined oral contraceptive for a short period (break)

For each description below, choose the **single** most appropriate answer from the above list of options. Each option may be used once, more than once, or not at all.

1 A 27-year-old woman presents with irregular vaginal bleeding of 4 months' duration. Her body mass index (BMI) is 30 and she has been on microgynon for the past 8 years without experiencing any problems. She has recently started a new relationship.

2 A 32-year-old woman attends the family planning clinic with irregular bleeding and spotting since Implanon was inserted 3 months ago. Her smear results have all been normal. She was on microgynon but switched to Implanon as she became more forgetful. She is very anxious as her mother died of cervical cancer at the age of 40.

3 A 27-year-old woman attends family planning clinic for advice. She is on the combined contraceptive pill and is comfortable with it. She has recently been diagnosed with seizures and been started on carbamazepine.

4 A 47-year-old lady attends the family planning clinic for advice. Her BMI is 36. She had a T-safe IUCD fitted 8 years ago. She has recently started to have intermenstrual bleeding and spotting. Her periods are regular. High vaginal and endocervical swabs arranged by her GP are negative. What is the appropriate management option?

5 A 36-year-old lady attends the gynaecology clinic for irregular bleeding per vaginum of 4 months' duration. She had Implanon fitted two and half years ago. She smokes about 20 cigarettes a day and has recently gained about 4 stone (25 kg). What is the appropriate option?

Answers: see page 146.

68 Termination of pregnancy

A vaginal prostaglandins
B pregnancy test
C ultrasound of the pelvis
D suction evacuation
E rectal metronidazole
F triple swabs
G oral misoprostol
H evacuation of retained products of conception
I involvement of social services
J repeating beta human chorionic gonadotrophin after 48 hours
K adoption
L an antibiotic course and repeat ultrasound
M laparoscopy and possible salpingectomy
N anti-D immunoglobulin
O mifepristone followed by gemeprost 48 hours later

For each description below, choose the **single** most appropriate answer from the above list of options. Each option may be used once, more than once, or not at all.

1 A 26-year-old lady attends the gynaecology clinic requesting termination of pregnancy (TOP). Her last menstrual period was 6 weeks ago. There is no history of abdominal pain or vaginal bleeding. She is in a stable relationship. What is the most appropriate option?

2 A 20-year-old girl attends the family planning walk-in clinic for a pregnancy test, which is positive. She is unsure of the date of her last menstrual period. She is a smoker and defaulted on her last depot contraceptive injection. She was treated for abdominal pain and discharge per vaginum last week. What is the most appropriate option?

3 A 19-year-old girl has been referred for TOP. Her last menstrual bleed was 5 months ago. Her periods are generally very regular. There was no bleeding or vaginal discharge. Her ultrasound shows an anencephalic fetus. What is the most appropriate method at this stage of gestation?

4 A 26-year-old woman underwent medical termination of pregnancy at 8 weeks' gestation. She then bled continuously for 3 weeks, for which a pelvic ultrasound was arranged by her GP. Ultrasound has shown a 50 × 20 mm retained product inside the uterine cavity. What is the next appropriate step in managing this scenario?

Answers: see page 147.

69 Sexually transmitted infections

A   azithromycin 2 g stat

B   pelvic ultrasound

C   laparoscopic drainage and parenteral antibiotics

D   contact tracing

E   test of cure

F   azithromycin 1 g stat

G   metronidazole 400 mg twice daily for 1 week

H   pregnancy test

I   intravenous cefoxitin and intravenous doxycycline followed by oral antibiotics

J   ciprofloxacin 500 mg oral single dose and referral to the genitourinary medicine clinic

K   laparoscopic adhesiolysis

L   removal of intrauterine contraceptive device (IUCD) and ofloxacin and metronidazole for 14 days

M   podophyllin ointment

N   steroid cream

O   electrocautery

P   removal of the IUCD

For each description below, choose the **single** most appropriate answer from the above list of options. Each option may be used once, more than once, or not at all.

1   A 27-year-old woman undergoes pre-IUCD insertion screening with triple swabs. She is asymptomatic and has been in a new relationship for the past 3 months. Her endocervical swabs show intracellular Gram-negative diplococci. What is the appropriate management option?

2   A 33-year-old woman is admitted to the gynaecology ward with abdominal pain and a swinging temperature. She was treated for vaginal discharge in a walk-in clinic, but details of the swab results are not available. On examination her temperature is 38.7°C with diffuse rigidity in the lower abdomen. A pregnancy test is negative. Ultrasound pelvis shows normal adnexa. What is the appropriate management option?

3   A 22-year-old woman attends the sexual health clinic with offensive vaginal discharge. She has been in a stable relationship for the past 4 years. Triple swabs are taken. Wet-mount examination shows motile flagellated protozoa. What is the appropriate management option?

4   A 28-year-old woman attends the emergency gynaecology clinic with vaginal discharge and abdominal pain. Her last menstrual period was 2 months ago, and

SEXUALLY TRANSMITTED INFECTIONS

an IUCD was fitted 3 months ago. She has been in a new relationship for the past 4 months. What is the appropriate management option?

5   A 38-year-old woman presents with vulval irritation and lumps in her vulva. On examination multiple keratinised warts are seen on the vulva. What is the appropriate management option?

Answers: see page 148.

ANSWERS

64 Human immunodeficiency virus infection

Answers: G I N M

A 21-year-old university student attends the genitourinary medicine (GUM) clinic requesting a sexually transmitted infection screen as her previous boyfriend has recently been diagnosed with human immunodeficiency virus (HIV) infection. She is completely asymptomatic and otherwise fit and healthy. She is found to be HIV positive. Her CD4 count is 1000 cells/mm³. Swabs for other sexually transmitted infections are negative. She is counselled fully about the diagnosis. What is the most suitable next step in her management?

G   Treatment is not indicated in asymptomatic patients with a CD4 cell count of greater than 350 cells/mm³.

A 28-year-old woman attends the GUM clinic. She is a known HIV-positive patient. Her most recent blood tests have shown normal liver function tests and a CD4 cell count of 500 cells/mm³. She is currently on GUM follow-up. She states that she is 6 months pregnant and has not so far had any antenatal checks. What is the most appropriate treatment option?

I   These interventions can reduce the risk of vertical transmission from 30 to 2 per cent.

A 36-year-old intravenous drug user attends the Accident and Emergency department with a dry cough and breathlessness. Her chest X-ray shows bilateral perihilar interstitial shadows. She was first diagnosed with HIV infection 2 years ago, and is being followed up with blood results. She has recently defaulted treatment. Her CD4 count is 100 cells/mm³. What is the best management option?

N   High-dose intravenous co-trimoxazole is the treatment of choice in *Pneumocystis carinii* pneumonia.

A 28-year-old woman is seen in the sexual health clinic for contraceptive advice. She was diagnosed with HIV infection 2 months ago. Her CD4 count is 800 cells/mm³. She is completely asymptomatic. What is the most appropriate method of contraception?

M   A barrier method of contraception is needed in addition to a reliable contraceptive method.

65 Choice of contraception

Answers: C B M I H

An 18-year-old girl requests contraception. She has been sexually active for 2 years and has been in a new relationship for the past 3 weeks. What is the most appropriate option?

C   Barrier methods provide protection against sexually transmitted diseases but have a higher failure rate. They should be used along with a reliable method, for example the combined oral contraceptive pill.

A 34-year-old lady requests contraception. Her body mass index (BMI) is 35. She suffers from painful heavy periods. She thinks she has completed her family. She smokes 10 cigarettes a day. What is the most appropriate option?

B   The Mirena coil is now licensed for the treatment for menorrhagia. It is also one of the long-acting reliable contraceptive methods, with a failure rate of 0–0.2 per HWY (hundred woman years).

A 29-year-old lady with a BMI of 37 who is para 4 is requesting permanent contraception. She fell pregnant on the combined oral contraceptive pill, and her periods are normal and last for 5 days. She had an intrauterine contraceptive device in the past and did not like it. She is worried about weight gain with Implanon and depot progesterone. What is the most appropriate option?

M   Vasectomy can be considered in this scenario. The failure rate of vasectomy is 1:2000, compared with female sterilization, with a rate of 1:200.

A 42-year-old lady who is para 3 requests contraception. She has been on the combined oral contraceptive pill for many years. She has recently become forgetful and requests an alternate non-hormonal long-term method. What is the most appropriate option?

I   All contraceptive methods are more reliable in this age group because of the age-related decline in fertility. A copper IUCD can be left for 10 years in women aged 40 and above.

A 26-year-old lady gave birth to a baby a month ago and is breast-feeding the baby. She was on the combined pill before and had no complaints with that. She has needle phobia and requests a short-term contraceptive. What is the most appropriate option?

H   All progestogen-only methods, such as the minipill, Depo-Provera, Implanon and Mirena intrauterine system, can be considered in breast-feeding women.

66 Emergency contraception

Answers: I H I L N

A 20-year-old girl attends the family planning clinic 6 hours after unprotected sexual intercourse. Her periods are regular and the first day of her last menstrual period was 3 weeks ago. Her current contraceptive method is male condoms. She also recalls another episode of condom split 10 days ago. Her pregnancy test is negative. What is the most appropriate advice?

I   There is no evidence for progesterone-only emergency contraception causing spontaneous miscarriage if the patient is already pregnant. However, the woman should be advised to return for a pregnancy test.

A 27-year-old lady attends the family planning clinic 7 days after unprotected sexual intercourse. Her menstrual cycles are very regular (K3–4/28). Her last menstrual period was 2 weeks ago. What is the most appropriate option?

H   A copper IUCD can be offered up to 5 days after ovulation if the woman has a regular 28-day cycle.

A 37-year-old woman attends the clinic 6 hours after unprotected sexual intercourse. She suffers from idiopathic thrombocytopenic purpura and is on long-term steroids. Her periods are regular but heavy, and the first day of her last menstrual period was 2 weeks ago. What is the most appropriate option?

I   Hormonal contraception is preferred to a copper coil as an IUCD might aggravate menorrhagia.

A 23-year-old nulliparous woman attends Accident and Emergency. She gives a history of unprotected sexual intercourse the previous night. Her periods are regular (3–4/30). She had sexual intercourse with a stranger. Her last menstrual period was 2 weeks ago. What is the most appropriate step?

L   Unprotected sexual intercourse carries a risk of sexually transmitted infections in addition to a risk of pregnancy.

A 19-year-old girl requests emergency contraception. She gives a history of unprotected sexual intercourse 40 hours ago. She is unsure of when her last menstrual period was as her periods are irregular. Her regular contraceptive method is the male condom. What is the first step in management?

N   A pregnancy test would be the most appropriate option. However, it could be negative in early pregnancy.

67 Contraception

Answers: E C G M E

A 27-year-old woman presents with irregular vaginal bleeding of 4 months' duration. Her body mass index (BMI) is 30 and she has been on microgynon for the past 8 years without experiencing any problems. She has recently started a new relationship.

E   Breakthrough bleeding in women previously well controlled with the combined pill may be a marker of sexually transmitted infection.

A 32-year-old woman attends the family planning clinic with irregular bleeding and spotting since Implanon was inserted 3 months ago. Her smear results have all been normal. She was on microgynon but switched to Implanon as she became more forgetful. She is very anxious as her mother died of cervical cancer at the age of 40.

C   Irregular bleeding and spotting is a known side-effect of progestogen-only methods and usually settles down within 3–6 months.

A 27-year-old woman attends family planning clinic for advice. She is on the combined contraceptive pill and is comfortable with it. She has recently been diagnosed with seizures and been started on carbamazepine.

G   Carbamazepine is an enzyme inducer, and other long-term reliable contraceptives should be offered.

A 47-year-old lady attends the family planning clinic for advice. Her BMI is 36. She had a T-safe IUCD fitted 8 years ago. She has recently started to have intermenstrual bleeding and spotting. Her periods are regular. High vaginal and endocervical swabs arranged by her GP are negative. What is the appropriate management option?

M   Perimenopausal bleeding needs to be evaluated after removal of the coil.

A 36-year-old lady attends the gynaecology clinic for irregular bleeding per vaginum of 4 months' duration. She had Implanon fitted two and half years ago. She smokes about 20 cigarettes a day and has recently gained about 4 stone (25 kg). What is the appropriate option?

E   Breakthrough bleeding in women could be a symptom of sexually transmitted infection and has to be ruled out.

68 Termination of pregnancy

Answers: O C O H

A 26-year-old lady attends the gynaecology clinic requesting termination of pregnancy (TOP). Her last menstrual period was 6 weeks ago. There is no history of abdominal pain or vaginal bleeding. She is in a stable relationship. What is the most appropriate option?

O   Medical termination with mifepristone plus prostaglandin could be offered for pregnancies of less than 9 weeks' duration.

A 20-year-old girl attends the family planning walk-in clinic for a pregnancy test, which is positive. She is unsure of the date of her last menstrual period. She is a smoker and defaulted on her last depot contraceptive injection. She was treated for abdominal pain and discharge per vaginum last week. What is the most appropriate option?

C   Pelvic ultrasound is appropriate where gestation is in doubt or extrauterine pregnancy is suspected.

A 19-year-old girl has been referred for TOP. Her last menstrual bleed was 5 months ago. Her periods are generally very regular. There was no bleeding or vaginal discharge. Her ultrasound shows an anencephalic fetus. What is the most appropriate method at this stage of gestation?

O   For a mid-trimester termination (13–24 weeks of gestation) medical termination with mifepristone followed by prostaglandin is an appropriate method and has been shown to be safe and effective. For the mid-trimester a dose of 200 mg mifepristone is adequate.

A 26-year-old woman underwent medical termination of pregnancy at 8 weeks' gestation. She then bled continuously for 3 weeks, for which a pelvic ultrasound was arranged by her GP. Ultrasound has shown a 50 × 20 mm retained product inside the uterine cavity. What is the next appropriate step in managing this scenario?

H   Persistence of placental or fetal tissue is more common following early medical termination, and up to 5 per cent of women require a surgical evacuation.

69 Sexually transmitted infections

Answers: J I G H O

A 27-year-old woman undergoes pre-IUCD insertion screening with triple swabs. She is asymptomatic and has been in a new relationship for the past 3 months. Her endocervical swabs show intracellular Gram-negative diplococci. What is the appropriate management option?

J   Ciprofloxacin 500 mg orally and ofloxacin 400 mg are both recommended treatment options for uncomplicated gonococcal infection.

A 33-year-old woman is admitted to the gynaecology ward with abdominal pain and a swinging temperature. She was treated for vaginal discharge in a walk-in clinic, but details of the swab results are not available. On examination her temperature is 38.7°C with diffuse rigidity in the lower abdomen. A pregnancy test is negative. Ultrasound pelvis shows normal adnexa. What is the appropriate management option?

I   Initial parenteral therapy followed by oral doxycycline 100 mg daily and metronidazole 400 mg twice daily is a recommended option in severe pelvic inflammatory disease.

A 22-year-old woman attends the sexual health clinic with offensive vaginal discharge. She has been in a stable relationship for the past 4 years. Triple swabs are taken. Wet-mount examination shows motile flagellated protozoa. What is the appropriate management option?

G   Oral metronidazole 2 g as a stat dose or 400 mg twice daily for a week are both accepted regimens for treating trichomonal infection.

A 28-year-old woman attends the emergency gynaecology clinic with vaginal discharge and abdominal pain. Her last menstrual period was 2 months ago, and an IUCD was fitted 3 months ago. She has been in a new relationship for the past 4 months. What is the appropriate management option?

H   Ectopic pregnancy is suspected whenever a possibly fertile woman has abdominal pain. Pregnancy test is the first line of investigation.

A 38-year-old woman presents with vulval irritation and lumps in her vulva. On examination multiple keratinised warts are seen on the vulva. What is the appropriate management option?

O   Ablative treatment techniques are generally recommended for keratinised warts.

Section 13: Early pregnancy complications

70 **Recurrent miscarriage**

71 **Management of bleeding in early pregnancy**

QUESTIONS

70 Recurrent miscarriage

A diabetes screening
B thyroid function tests
C progestogen supplementation
D chorionic gonadotrophin
E serum prolactin level
F prednisolone therapy
G glucose tolerance test and thyroid function tests
H parental karyotype, thrombophilia screening and pelvic ultrasound
I aspirin and heparin during pregnancy
J immunotherapy
K TORCH (toxoplasmosis, rubella, cytomegalovirus, herpes simplex and human immunodeficiency virus) screen, karyotyping + APS (antiphospholipid syndrome), ACL (anticardiolipin antibody)
L treatment of bacterial vaginosis
M reassurance
N cervical cerclage
O aspirin during pregnancy

For each description below, choose the **single** most appropriate answer from the above list of options. Each option may be used once, more than once, or not at all.

1 A 28 year-old-lady attends the gynaecology clinic after three consecutive miscarriages. She and her partner are otherwise well and anxious to start a family. What is the most appropriate advice?

2 A 28-year-old lady presents with her partner after two consecutive miscarriages. Her last two miscarriages were in the middle trimester. She complains of a greyish discharge and her pregnancy test is positive.

3 A 28-year-old lady presents with a positive pregnancy test in her fourth pregnancy at 7 weeks. She has had three consecutive miscarriages. Her blood results have shown anticardiolipin antibodies on two occasions.

4 A 28-year-old lady presents in her fourth pregnancy at 14 weeks. Her three miscarriages were in the middle trimester. On examination the cervix is found to be 2 cm dilated with coning of the membranes on ultrasound.

5 A couple are seen in the gynaecology clinic after their third miscarriage. The karyotyping is normal. Thrombophilia screening is negative. Pelvic ultrasound is normal.

Answers: see page 152.

71 Management of bleeding in early pregnancy

A elective evacuation of retained products of conception
B repeat ultrasound scan in 10–14 days
C reassurance and discharge
D medical management with mifepristone/misoprostol
E intravenous access, fluid replacement and urgent curettage
F laparoscopy and salpingectomy
G laparotomy
H repeat ultrasound in 4 days
I folic acid
J serial beta human chorionic gonadotrophin (bhCG) measurement
K culdocentesis
L diagnostic curettage to look for chorionic villi
M conservative management
N referral to an appropriate centre
O transvaginal ultrasound

For each description below, choose the **single** most appropriate answer from the above list of options. Each option may be used once, more than once, or not at all.

1 A 36-year-old lady who is para 2 presents at 10 week's gestation with excessive bleeding and feeling cold and clammy. She is tachycardic on admission with a heart rate of 120 beats/minute. On examination the os is open.

2 A nulliparous 21-year-old lady presents with abdominal pain occurring for the past 4 hours. She gives a history of fainting. She has a positive pregnancy test. She has irregular periods and cannot recall the date of her last menstrual period. Ultrasound shows a thick endometrium with no fetal pole within the uterus. There is a small amount of free fluid in POD (Pouch of Douglas). She complains of left adnexal pain and has signs of peritonism. She is tachycardic and has a normal blood pressure. Serum bhCG (beta human chorionic gonadotrophin) is 2300 IU and haemoglobin level is 95 g/dL.

3 A 31-year-old woman presents with bleeding per vaginum. She is unsure of the date of her last menstrual period. On ultrasound there is an intrauterine gestational sac 17 mm in size with no contents.

4 A 27-year-old woman presents with history of bleeding at 8 weeks' gestation. Ultrasound shows a viable intrauterine pregnancy of 7 weeks' gestation. There is an 18 × 20 mm subchorionic haematoma. On examination there is no active bleeding.

5 A 31-year-old lady attends for a nuchal translucency scan at 11 weeks' gestation. She is found to have a gestational sac of 23 mm with a yolk sac. No fetal pole is recognised.

Answers: see page 152.

ANSWERS

70 Recurrent miscarriage

Answers: H L I N M

A 28 year-old-lady attends the gynaecology clinic after three consecutive miscarriages. She and her partner are otherwise well and anxious to start a family. What is the most appropriate advice?

H   This is the standard set of tests needed for recurrent miscarriage.

A 28-year-old lady presents with her partner after two consecutive miscarriages. Her last two miscarriages were in the middle trimester. She complains of a greyish discharge and her pregnancy test is positive.

L   Treatment of bacterial vaginosis improves outcome in women with a previous second-trimester miscarriage.

A 28-year-old lady presents with a positive pregnancy test in her fourth pregnancy at 7 weeks. She has had three consecutive miscarriages. Her blood results have shown anticardiolipin antibodies on two occasions.

I   The presence of anticardiolipin/antiphospholipid is associated with a better outcome if treated with aspirin and heparin rather than aspirin alone.

A 28-year-old lady presents in her fourth pregnancy at 14 weeks. Her three miscarriages were in the middle trimester. On examination the cervix is found to be 2 cm dilated with coning of the membranes on ultrasound.

N   Cervical incompetence probably benefits from a 'rescue' cerclage. The use of prophylactic cerclage is debatable.

A couple are seen in the gynaecology clinic after their third miscarriage. The karyotyping is normal. Thrombophilia screening is negative. Pelvic ultrasound is normal.

M   Normal investigations imply an unexplained recurrent miscarriage. This has a subsequent 75 per cent chance of a successful future pregnancy.

71 Management of bleeding in early pregnancy

Answers: E F B C A

A 36-year-old lady who is para 2 presents at 10 week's gestation with excessive bleeding and feeling cold and clammy. She is tachycardic on admission with a heart rate of 120 beats/minute. On examination the os is open.

E   Urgent curettage is needed in incomplete miscarriage with heavy bleeding and clinical signs of cardiac compensation.

A nulliparous 21-year-old lady presents with abdominal pain occurring for the past 4 hours. She gives a history of fainting. She has a positive pregnancy test. She has irregular periods and cannot recall the date of her last menstrual period. Ultrasound shows a thick endometrium with no fetal pole within the uterus. There is a small amount of free fluid in POD (Pouch of Douglas). She complains of left

adnexal pain and has signs of peritonism. She is tachycardic and has a normal blood pressure. Serum bhCG (beta human chorionic gonadotrophin) is 2300 IU and haemoglobin level is 95 g/dL.

F Laparoscopy with or without salpingectomy is necessary for suspected ectopic pregnancy. Conservative management is not indicated here as the woman has signs of internal haemorrhage. The procedure can be performed laparoscopically if the surgeon is competent as the woman's haemoglobin level is not excessively low.

A 31-year-old woman presents with bleeding per vaginum. She is unsure of the date of her last menstrual period. On ultrasound there is an intrauterine gestational sac 17 mm in size with no contents.

B A sac size of 20 mm is a minimal requirement for the diagnosis of failed intrauterine pregnancy.

A 27-year-old woman presents with history of bleeding at 8 weeks' gestation. Ultrasound shows a viable intrauterine pregnancy of 7 weeks' gestation. There is an 18 × 20 mm subchorionic haematoma. On examination there is no active bleeding.

C Subchorionic haematoma has no adverse effect on the outcome of pregnancy in the absence of bleeding. Over 90 per cent of women have a positive pregnancy outcome.

A 31-year-old lady attends for a nuchal translucency scan at 11 weeks' gestation. She is found to have a gestational sac of 23 mm with a yolk sac. No fetal pole is recognised.

A A sac size of more than 20 mm with no fetal pole is diagnostic of anembryonic pregnancy. Elective curettage is often needed.

Index

Note: References are to the question and answer number and not the page number.

abdominal hysterectomy 43, 55
  adnexal masses 62
  caesarean 3
  colposcopy indicating 51
  endometrial cancer 47
  endometriosis 55, 63
  postoperative investigations 52
abdominal pain in pregnancy
  diagnosis 12
  management 11
abdominoperineal septal resection 42
abortion
  spontaneous *see* miscarriage
  therapeutic 68
    under-16 year olds 2
accelerations, absence 26
adnexal masses 50, 62
adolescent amenorrhoea 42, 46, 58
adrenal hyperplasia, congenital 46
  late-onset 58
adrenaline 1
advanced life support 1
airway/breathing/circulation, CS 4
alcoholism 12
amenorrhoea 58
  adolescent 42, 46, 58
amniotic fluid embolism 25, 27
anaesthesia
  examination under, postmenopausal
    bleeding 61
  obstetric 4
anal sphincter repair 32
analgesics
  fibroids 40
  opioid, constipation 11
anaphylactic shock 1
androgen insensitivity syndrome, complete
    and partial 46
anembryonic pregnancy 71

anovulation 57
antenatal care 36–8
antibiotics
  bacterial vaginosis 31
  P. carinii pneumonia 64
  preterm premature rupture of
    membranes 31
  pyelonephritis 11
  STDs 69
antiphospholipid syndrome 70
antiretroviral drugs 9
  highly-active (HAART) 64
antithyroid drugs 16
aortic dissection 17
appendicitis 12
asthenospermia and oligospermia 57
atonic postpartum haemorrhage 25
atosiban 31
atrial fibrillation 19
atrophic vaginitis 61
azoospermia 56

bacterial vaginosis 31, 70
barrier contraception and STDs 65
  HIV 64
bereavement counselling 30
bile acids, serum 10
biliary disease 10, 11, 20
bimanual compression 29
biopsy
  colposcopy-directed 51
  endometrial 43, 61
bladder
  iatrogenic damage/injury 54
    in CS 3
  outflow obstruction 59
  see also cystocele; vesicovaginal fistula
bleeding *see* haemorrhage
blood patch, epidural 4

blood sampling, fetal 26
bowel
  damage
    in CS 3
    in vaginal delivery 32
  disease in pregnancy 13
brachytherapy, cervical cancer 48
brain tumour 23
breast cancer 6
  oestrogen receptor-positive 63
  tamoxifen 61
breast-feeding and HIV 9, 64
breech presentation 33
  persistent 34
brow presentation 34

caesarean section (CS) 3, 4
  in fetal death 30
  HIV and 9, 64
  malpresentations indicating 33
  previous, trial of labour 34
cancer 47–51
  breast see breast cancer
  cervical 48, 51, 59
  ovarian, postoperative complications 54
carbamazepine and combined oral
    contraceptives 67
carboprost, intramuscular 29
cardiac disease see heart disease
cardiotocography (CTG)
  in cholestasis 10
  intrapartum 26
CD4 cell count, monitoring 64
cephalic version, external 33
cervix
  cancer 48, 51, 59
  incompetence 70
  intraepithelial neoplasia (CIN) 51
  screening 44
  smear see smear
  trauma 25
  see also colposcopy
chancroid 39
chemotherapy
  breast cancer 6
  cervical cancer 48, 51
  endometrial cancer 47
  trophoblastic disease 45
chest pain 17
chest tube insertion 1
childbirth, smear test after 44
children
  gynaecological conditions 46
  medicolegal issues 2
  see also adolescent; neonates

cholecystectomy, laparoscopic 11
cholestasis, obstetric 10, 20
chromosomal abnormalities,
    antenatal 36
clomiphene-resistant anovulation 56
clotting screen 35
cluster headache 23
coagulation (clotting) screen 35
colitis, ulcerative 13
collapse, maternal 27
colostomy, defunctioning 32
colporrhaphy, posterior 41
colposcopy 44, 51
combined oral contraceptive pill 43, 67
  HIV and 64
complications
  3rd stage of labour 25
  postoperative, management 53
    late 55
  pregnancy 6–23
compression stockings 14
condom, combined oral contraceptive and
    (double Dutch method) 65
  HIV 64
congenital adrenal hyperplasia see adrenal
    hyperplasia
congenital Müllerian anomalies 42
constipation, opioids 11
contraception 65–7
  emergency 65, 66
  STDs and 64, 65
convulsion (fit), eclamptic 27
copper IUCD 66
cord prolapse 34
coronary heart disease 17
corticosteroids see steroids
cotrimoxazole 9
counselling
  intrauterine death 30
  irregular bleeding with Implanon 67
  Müllerian defects 42
Crohn's disease 13
cyst, ovarian see ovaries
cystic fibrosis 37
cystocele 60
cytogenetic abnormalities, antenatal 36

de Quervain's thyroiditis 16
death, intrauterine 30
decelerations
  persistent late 26
  variable and early 26
delivery 24
  cancer treatment deferred until after 6
  in fetal death 30

delivery room management 5
depression 21, 22
dexamethasone, preterm labour 31
diabetes mellitus 18, 27
dizziness 15
double Dutch method *see* condom
Down's syndrome 36
drugs in pregnancy 21

eclamptic fit 27
ectopic (extrauterine) pregnancy 68,
    69, 71
Edwards' syndrome 36
egg (ovum) donation 56
embolism
    amniotic fluid 25, 27
    pulmonary 35
emergency contraception 65, 66
emesis 20
endometrial cancer, omentectomy 47
endometriosis 55, 57
    surgery 56, 63
endometrium
    biopsy 43, 61
    cancer 47
    polypectomy 61
enoxaparin 14
epidural blood patch 4
epinephrine (adrenaline) 1
erythromycin, preterm premature rupture
    of membranes 31
evacuation and curettage
    retained products of conception 68
    trophoblastic disease 45
extension (in delivery) 24
external cephalic version 33

face presentation 34
fallopian tubes
    complete absence 42
    in subfertility causation 57
    see also salpingo-oophorectomy
fatty liver 12, 20
fertility problems *see* subfertility
fetus
    death 30
    growth restriction 36
    thyrotoxicosis 16
    well-being assessment 1
        intrapartum 26
fibroids 38, 40, 55
fistula, vesicovaginal 59
fit, eclamptic 27
flexion (in delivery) 24

fluid management
    fibroids 40
    resuscitation 1
    sickle cell crisis 11
folic acid 9
footling breech presentation 33
forceps delivery 5
fresh frozen plasma, postpartum
    haemorrhage 29

gallstones 11, 12, 20
gas induction of anaesthesia 4
gastrointestinal tract
    damage in CS 3
    disorders 13
gemeprost, therapeutic termination 68
genetics 37
    see also cytogenetic abnormalities
genital herpes 39
gestational trophoblastic disease 38, 45
Gillick/Fraser competency 2
glucose tolerance test 18
gonadotrophin-releasing hormone (GnRH)
    analogue, fibroids 40
gonorrhoea 69
Graves' disease 16
growth restriction, intrauterine 36

haemoglobin, glycosylated 18
haemorrhage/bleeding
    early pregnancy 71
    with hormonal contraceptives 67
    postmenopausal 61
    postpartum 29
        atonic 25
    subarachnoid 27
haemorroids, prolapsed 13
headache 23
heart disease
    ischaemic *see* ischaemic heart disease
    rheumatic 19
HELPP syndrome 35
heparin (incl. LMW heparin) 14
hepatitis, viral 20
    HBV
        neonatal vaccination 7
        vertical transmission 8
    HCV, vertical transmission 8
herpes genitalis 39
herpes zoster 7
HIV 9, 64
    vertical transmission 8, 64
hormone replacement therapy (HRT)
    62–3
    endometriosis and 55

human immunodeficiency virus *see* HIV
11-β-hydroxylase deficiency 46
hyperemesis gravidarum 20
hypoglycaemia 27
hypotension, supine 15
hysterectomy
   abdominal *see* abdominal hysterectomy
   cervical cancer 48
   endometrial cancer 47
   endometriosis 55, 63
   postoperative investigations 52
   vaginal *see* vaginal hysterectomy
hysteroscopy 43
   postmenopausal bleeding 61

iatrogenic headache 23
iatrogenic injury
   CS 3
   gynaecological surgery, urinary tract 54
immunisation
   active, neonatal hepatitis B 7
   passive, varicella-zoster 7
Implanon 67
in vitro fertilisation (IVF) 56
incontinence, stress 55, 59, 60
induction of anaesthesia, gas 4
infections
   maternal 7
      vertical transmission 8
   sexually-transmitted *see* sexually-
      transmitted infections
infertility *see* subfertility
injury *see* trauma
instrumented delivery 5
insulin-dependent diabetes 18, 27
insulin therapy 18
intestine *see* bowel
intracranial haemorrhage 27
intracytoplasmic sperm injection (ICSI) 56
intraepithelial neoplasia, cervical (CIN) 51
intrauterine (contraceptive) device (IUD;
      IUCD) 67
   copper 66
   levonorgestrel-releasing 43, 65
intrauterine death 30
intrauterine growth restriction 36
intravenous access
   postpartum haemorrhage 29
   resuscitation 1
intravenous fluids *see* fluid management
ischaemic (coronary) heart disease 17
   HRT and 63
IU(C)D *see* intrauterine device

keratinised warts 69

labour 24–35
   3rd stage complications 25
   mechanism 24
   preterm *see* preterm labour
   risks 34
   trial of, with previous CS 34
labour suite, tests 35
labyrinthitis 15
laparoscopic procedures
   cholecystectomy 11
   endometriosis ablation 56
   ovarian cystectomy 50, 56
   ovarian drilling 56
laparotomy
   endometrial cancer 47
   ovarian cyst 50
large loop excision of transformation zone
      (LLETZ) 48, 51
legal issues 2
leiomyoma (fibroids) 38, 40, 55
levonorgestrel-releasing IUD 43, 65
levonorgestrel tablets 66
lichen sclerosus 49, 62
life support, advanced 1
liver
   fatty 12, 20
   function tests 20
lymphadenectomy (abdominopelvic)
   endometrial cancer 47
   vulval cancer 49

McRoberts manoeuvre 28
males
   condom *see* condom
   sterilisation 65
   subfertility 56, 57
malignancy *see* cancer
malpresentations 33, 34
medications in pregnancy 21
medicolegal issues 2
men *see* males
menopause 61–3
   HRT 62–3
   premature 56, 63
menorrhagia 43
mental health disorders 21, 22
methyldopa 21
metronidazole
   bacterial vaginosis 31
   trichomoniasis 69
Microgynon 67

mifepristone 68
minipill 65
Mirena 43, 65
miscarriage (failed pregnancy) 71
 incomplete 71
 recurrent 70
misoprostol 30
molar pregnancy 45
mortality, intrauterine 30
Müllerian defects 42
multiple pregnancy 38

Neisseria gonorrhoeae 69
neoadjuvant (preoperative) radiotherapy,
 vulval cancer 49
neonates
 hepatitis B vaccination 7
 thyrotoxicosis 16
 varicella-zoster Ig 7
neoplasms *see* cancer; tumours
neurological disorders 23
newborns *see* neonates
nifedipine 21, 23

oestrogen(s), local/topical
 postmenopausal bleeding 61
 uterovaginal prolapse 41
 see also combined oral contraceptive pill;
 hormone replacement therapy
oestrogen receptor-positive breast
 cancer 63
oligospermia 56
 and asthenospermia 57
omentectomy, endometrial cancer 47
oncology *see* cancer
oocyte (ovum) donation 56
oophorectomy *see* salpingo-oophorectomy
operative obstetrics 3–5
opioids, constipation 11
oral contraceptive pill
 combined *see* combined oral
 contraceptive pill
 combining condom with *see* condom
 progestogen-only 65
osteoporosis 63
ovaries
 cancer, postoperative complications 54
 cyst
 management 50, 52, 56
 torsion (intrapartum) 25
 laparoscopic drilling 56
 polycystic ovarian syndrome 57, 58
 see also salpingo-oophorectomy

ovulatory failure 57
ovum donation 56

paediatrics *see* children; neonates
pain
 abdominal *see* abdominal pain
 chest 17
 see also analgesics; headache
palliative care
 cervical cancer 48, 51
 endometrial cancer 47
palpitations 19
pancreatitis 12, 20
pelvic floor exercises 41
pelvic floor repair, vaginal hysterectomy
 with 41, 55
pelvic inflammatory disease 69
pelvic lymphadenectomy *see*
 lymphadenectomy
pelvic manoeuvre 28
pelvic ultrasound *see* ultrasound
pericardial effusion 17
perineal injuries 32
peritoneal cytology, endometrial cancer 47
phaeochromocytoma 19
phenylephrine 4
phenytoin 21
placenta praevia 3
placental abruption 1
plasma, fresh frozen, postpartum
 haemorrhage 29
pneumonia 9, 17
 Pneumocystis carinii 9, 64
pneumothorax, tension 1
police 2
polycystic ovarian syndrome 57, 58
polyhydramnios 38
polypectomy, endometrial 61
postmenopausal bleeding 61
postpartum period (puerperium)
 haemorrhage *see* haemorrhage
 psychosis 22
 smear test 44
 thyroiditis 16
post-traumatic stress disorder 22
pregnancy
 anembryonic 71
 bleeding in early stages 71
 extrauterine/ectopic 68, 69, 71
 failed *see* miscarriage
 HIV and 9, 64
 loss *see* abortion; death; miscarriage
 medical complications 6–23

pregnancy (*Contd*)
 medications in 21
 molar 45
 multiple 38
pregnancy test 2, 58, 66, 69
premature labour *see* preterm labour
premature menopause 56, 63
premature rupture of membranes,
  preterm 31
prenatal care 36–8
preoperative radiotherapy, vulval cancer 49
presentation abnormalities 33, 34
preterm labour 31
 diagnosis 35
 steroids 10, 31
preterm premature rupture of
  membranes 31
progestogen-only implant (Implanon) 67
progestogen-only pill 65
progestogen-releasing (levonorgestrel-
  releasing) IUD 43, 65
prostaglandin, vaginal
 fetal death 30
 therapeutic termination 68
psychiatric disorders 21, 22
psychosexual counselling, Müllerian
  defects 42
psychosis, puerperal 22
puerperium *see* postpartum period
pulmonary embolism 35
pyelonephritis 11, 12

radiotherapy
 breast cancer 6
 cervical cancer 48, 51
 endometrial cancer 47
 vulval cancer, preoperative 49
rectal mucosal defect repair 32
restitution 24
resuscitation 1
retained products of conception,
  evacuation 68
rheumatic heart disease 19
ring pessary 41
rupture of membranes, preterm
  premature 31

sacrocolpopexy, open 41
salpingo-oophorectomy, bilateral,
  abdominal hysterectomy and
 adnexal masses 62
 endometrial cancer 47
 endometriosis 55, 63

scalp electrode, fetal 26
screening
 antenatal 36
 cervical 44
  see also smear
seizure (fit), eclamptic 27
sexual health 64–9
sexually-transmitted infections (STIs/STDs)
  39, 69
 barrier contraception *see* barrier
  contraception
shingles 7
shoulder dystocia 28
sickle cell crisis 11
small bowel damage in CS 3
smear, cervical
 annual 48
 postpartum 44
sperm abnormalities 56, 57
sterilisation, male 65
steroids
 lichen sclerosus 49, 62
 preterm labour 10, 31
stress incontinence 55, 59, 60
subarachnoid haemorrhage 27
subfertility 56–8
 causes 57
 management 56
supine hypotension 15
suprapubic pressure 28
surgery 52–5
 cervical cancer 48
 endometrial cancer 47
 endometriosis 56, 63
 obstetric 3–5
 ovarian cyst 50, 56
 postoperative complications *see*
  complications
 postoperative investigations 52
 vulval cancer 49
 see also specific procedures
syncope 15
syphilis 39

tamoxifen 61
tension-free vaginal tape 55, 60
tension headache 23
tension pneumothorax 1
thromboembolism 14
 see also embolism
thyroid diseases 16
thyroiditis 16

thyrotoxicosis
  fetal/neonatal 16
  maternal 19
tocolytic 31
trachelectomy 48
transformation zone, large loop excision
  (LLETZ) 48, 51
trauma 2
  advanced life support 1
  iatrogenic *see* iatrogenic injury
  intrapartum 25, 32
trichomoniasis 69
triploidy 36
trisomy 18 (Edwards' syndrome) 36
trisomy 21 (Down's syndrome) 36
trophoblastic disease 38, 45
tumours
  brain 23
  malignant *see* cancer
Turner's syndrome 46, 58
twins or multiple pregnancy 38

ulcer(s), vulval 39
ulcerative colitis 13
ultrasound
  abdominopelvic
    ovarian cyst 50
    pregnancy diagnosis 68
  breast cancer 6
ultrasound-guided aspiration of pelvic
  collection 55
umbilical cord prolapse 34
ureter, iatrogenic injury 54
urinary tract 59–60
  iatrogenic injuries 54
urine culture 11
urodynamic stress incontinence 59, 60
uterovaginal prolapse 41
uterus
  bicornuate 42
  complete absence 42
  fibroids 38, 40, 55
  neck of *see* cervix
  retroversion/incarceration 59

vaccination, neonatal hepatitis B 7
vacuum (ventouse) delivery 5, 26
vagina
  fistula between bladder and 59
  prolapse 41
  prostaglandin application *see*
    prostaglandin
  septum 42
vaginal hysterectomy
  with pelvic floor repair 41, 55
  postoperative investigations 52
vaginal tape, tension-free 55, 60
vaginitis, atrophic 61
vaginoplasty 42
vaginosis, bacterial 31, 70
varicella-zoster Ig
  maternal 7
  neonatal 7
vasa praevia 35
vasectomy 65
vasovagal attack 15
venous disorders (incl. thromboembolism)
  14
  see also embolism
ventouse delivery 5, 26
vertigo 15
vesicovaginal fistula 59
vestibulitis, vulval 39
viral hepatitis *see* hepatitis
vitamin K 10
vomiting 20
vulva
  carcinoma 49
  keratinised warts 69
  lichen sclerosus 49, 62
  ulcers 39

warts, keratinised 69
weight reduction
  stress incontinence 60
  subfertility 56

Zavanelli's technique 28
zoster (shingles) 7

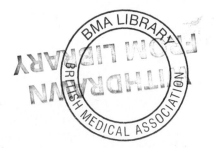